SUICIDE AND HOMICIDE AMONG ADOLESCENTS

Suicide and Homicide among Adolescents

PAUL C. HOLINGER, M.D., M.P.H.
DANIEL OFFER, M.D.
JAMES T. BARTER, M.D.
CARL C. BELL, M.D.

THE GUILFORD PRESS
New York   London

© 1994 The Guilford Press
A Division of Guilford Publications, Inc.
72 Spring Street, New York, NY 10012

Printed in the United States of America

This book is printed on acid-free paper.

Last digit is print number: 9   8   7   6   5   4   3   2

Library of Congress Cataloging-in-Publication Data

Suicide and homicide among adolescents / Paul C. Holinger . . . [et
al.].
        p.   cm.
    Includes bibliographical references and index.
    ISBN 0-89862-788-5
    1. Teenagers—Suicidal behavior. 2. Juvenile homicide.
3. Psychiatric epidemiology. I. Holinger, Paul C.
    [DNLM: 1. Suicide—in adolescence. 2. Homicide—in adolescence.
HV 6546 S9479 1994]
HF6546.S833   1994
362.2'8'0835—dc20
DNLM/DLC
for Library of Congress   93-50150
                                                              CIP

Acknowledgments

This study has taken years to complete, and we are very grateful to the many individuals who helped along the way. We thank the following for their various and essential contributions: Mr. Willie Cade, Chief, Productancy Inc. (for the design and execution of the graphs and Appendices); Dr. David Clark, Director, Center for Suicide Research and Prevention, Rush–Presbyterian–St. Luke's Medical Center (for overall direction and much of Chapter 1); Mr. Bruce Briscoe, Department of Psychology, Northwestern University, and Dr. Kenneth I. Howard, Professor of Psychology, Northwestern University (for statistical analysis); Ms. Laura G. Andersen and Ms. Betty Melton and her staff (for logistical and technical assistance); and Mr. Seymour Weingarten, Editor-in-Chief, and Ms. Judith Grauman, Editorial Supervisor, of The Guilford Press (for years of encouragement and guidance on this project).

In addition, a number of colleagues gave us valuable assistance over the years of this project, and we would like to express our deep gratitude to them: Drs. Stacie Barkin, Carolyn R. Block, Pamela C. Cantor, Jan A. Fawcett, Herbert Hendin, Esther Jenkins, Douglass S. Judson, Gerald L. Klerman, Sheron Lawson, Kevin W. Luke, Paul Montes III, Sonia Perez, Cynthia Pfeffer, Susan Quigley, Mark L. Rosenberg, Toby Sadkin, Jay Sandlow, Howard S. Sudak, and Graciela Val.

Contents

SUICIDE AND HOMICIDE
AMONG ADOLESCENTS

CHAPTER ONE

Introduction

Chapter 1 introduces the purposes of this book, which include the integration of epidemiologic and clinical approaches to better understand youth suicide and homicide; the presentation of the epidemiologic patterns of suicide and homicide among youth in the United States and comparisons of those patterns with trends in other countries; the exploration of etiologic and treatment aspects of youth suicide and homicide from clinical perspectives; and the utilization of epidemiologic and clinical approaches in order to develop effective prevention and intervention strategies.

There are few more complex behaviors than suicide or homicide. The student must steep himself or herself in the diverse sciences of psychopathology, personality, psychodynamics, medicine, genetics, biochemistry and toxicology, psychopharmacology, psychotherapy, epidemiology, anthropology, sociology, and history simply to follow the relevant research that has been generated, let alone to make new contributions to existing knowledge. Scientific training in research implementation, analysis, and interpretation is fundamental to scientific thinking and clinical activity. In this day and age, it sometimes seems wrong to ask, "What scientific evidence guides this particular suicide intervention or prevention program?", and even more heretical to ask, "What scientific evidence supports the efficacy of this particular intervention program?" But the truth is that scientists and clinicians do not know enough about why people kill and are killed—and they know even less about how to stop people from doing so in significant numbers. The accumulated scientific knowledge about suicidal and homicidal behavior amounts to a modest thimbleful. What we need is more accurate and reliable knowledge to guide clinical thinking and interventions, if suicide and homicide are to be prevented on any large scale. This conclusion reflects the way things are in the field and the distance yet to be traveled. For example, despite the advent of the community mental health movement, modern biological psychiatry, and community-based crisis intervention programs, the U.S. suicide rate has tended to *climb* since the mid-1950s, and the U.S. homicide rate has tended to remain high following the increases beginning in the early 1960s (see Figure 1.1). In other words, clinicians working with extremely difficult patients and communities occasionally lose patients to suicide and homicide, despite their best efforts.

What can clinicians and other mental health workers do while waiting for the knowledge base to become more substantial? They can follow and study new research about suicidal and homicidal behavior. "Suicidology," or the study of suicidal behavior, is an interdisciplinary scientific discipline whose roots began with Durkheim (1897/1951) almost a century ago and whose emergence was signaled by the appearance of empirical, clinically guided studies such as those by Dahlgren (1945) and Stengel and Cook (1958). In the United States, suicide became a legitimate field of study with the seminal work of Robins and colleagues (1959) in St. Louis, Dorpat and Ripley (1960) in Seattle, and the founding fathers of the Los Angeles Suicide Prevention Center: Robert Litman, Edwin Shneidman, and Norman Farberow (Litman et al., 1963). Augmented by important contributions from Robins and Murphy in St. Louis and from the Los Angeles group, both the amount and the quality of suicide-related research have grown steadily over the last 30 years. The scientific study of homicide—those who are killed, as well as the perpetrators—appears to have a more recent and less substantial history than does the study of suicide. However, early work by Wolfgang (1958, 1959, 1968; Wolfgang and Ferracuti, 1967), and subsequent contributions over the past three decades by researchers such as Benedek (Benedek and

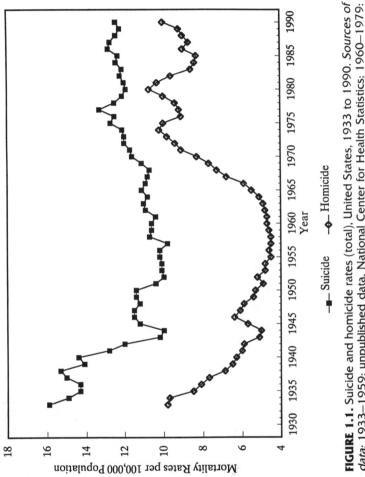

FIGURE 1.1. Suicide and homicide rates (total), United States, 1933 to 1990. *Sources of data:* 1933–1959: unpublished data, National Center for Health Statistics; 1960–1979: *Vital Statistics of the United States* (National Center for Health Statistics, 1964–1983); 1980–1990: unpublished data, National Center for Health Statistics.

3

Cornell, 1989), Block (1986, 1993), Christoffel (1990, 1991), Gelles (1987), Lewis et al. (1985), and others, have enhanced an understanding of the many facets of homicide. Despite the incompleteness of current knowledge about suicide and homicide, important facts and lessons can be discerned from study of the existing clinical and epidemiologic research. This volume on youth suicide and homicide attempts to review and integrate epidemiologic and clinical studies, for the purpose of achieving a better understanding of the phenomena of suicide and homicide.

INTEGRATING AN UNDERSTANDING OF YOUTH SUICIDE AND HOMICIDE

Although much has been written recently on youth suicide, and to a lesser extent on youth homicide, there have been relatively few efforts to compare, contrast, and integrate the phenomena of youthful suicide and homicide. Are there psychologic commonalities between murder of the other and murder of the self? Is the risk of violence equally likely to be expressed as suicide or homicide in certain individuals, depending on the situational circumstances?

The similarity of mortality patterns for suicide and homicide among youth suggests that these problems may be related in an epidemiologic sense, and that exploring them together may be useful. It is possible that these two forms of violent death share some common antecedents. It is also possible that public health policies or prevention strategies that reduce one cause of death may have value for reducing the other—as was suggested by a recent study showing that the imposition of strict gun control laws in Washington, D.C. reduced *both* suicide and homicide rates by about 25% (Loftin et al., 1991).

The phenomena of suicide and homicide may be related in a clinical sense as well. Though the rate of murder followed by suicide is relatively rare (averaging about 0.20–0.30 per 100,000 persons annually), murder or attempted murder followed by suicide accounts for about 5% of all homicidal deaths and about 1.5% of all suicidal deaths in the United States each year (Marzuk et al., 1992a; Palmer and Humphrey, 1980; Rosenbaum, 1990). In one of the early investigations of murder–suicide, Wolfgang (1958) studied 588 consecutive criminal homicides implicating 621 perpetrators in Philadelphia between 1948 and 1952. Four percent of the 621 later killed themselves.

INTEGRATING EPIDEMIOLOGIC AND CLINICAL VIEWPOINTS

This book also attempts to integrate the epidemiologic and clinical frames of reference in the areas of youth suicide and homicide. An understanding of the prevention and treatment of youth violence is enhanced by advances in the epidemiologic arena, just as epidemiologic understanding can benefit from clinical knowledge.

What value does the epidemiologic point of view hold for clinicians? Epidemiologic data help clarify the degree to which such problems as suicide and homicide vary by country and culture, sex, race/ethnicity, age, marital status, work status, and psychiatric status. In turn, this information helps us understand some of the ecologic forces that modify suicide and homicide risk, and helps us identify high-risk groups for clinical intervention and clinical research.

Epidemiologic studies also help correct misimpressions that arise from and are perpetuated in clinical practice. For example, experience with a wide range of suicidal patients has led many clinicians to postulate the existence of a "continuum of suicidal behavior," which assumes that persons with no history of suicidal thoughts, those having suicidal ideation, those who have made mild to severe suicide attempts, and those who have died by suicide can be classified meaningfully on a single underlying continuum of "suicidality." With the introduction of standardized epidemiologic studies, however, important qualitative differences between suicide completers and suicide attempters have become increasingly apparent. There is some overlap between the two

groups, but that overlap is apparently small. Long-term follow-up studies of persons who have made nonfatal suicide
attempts show that only 7%–10% eventually die by suicide
(Ettlinger, 1964; Motto, 1965; Weiss and Scott, 1974; Cullberg et al., 1988). Men die by suicide three to four times
more often than women, but women make nonfatal attempts
three to four times more often than men (Murphy, 1986).
Prevalence rates of major psychiatric disorder are much
higher among suicide completers, and prevalence rates of
personality disorder are much higher among those making
nonfatal attempts (Murphy, 1986). Living conditions, social
circumstances, and acute life traumas appear to play a much
greater role in the shaping of nonfatal attempts than of
death by suicide (Robins, 1986; Murphy, 1986). The appropriate conclusion to draw from these epidemiologic studies is
one of caution about generalizing from those making nonfatal attempts (with whom the clinician may be more familiar)
to those who die by suicide. Most of our clinical knowledge
about suicidal behavior is based on studies of ideators and
attempters, because these patients are accessible to study.
However, increasing evidence shows that the profiles of persons who make nonlethal attempts are very different from
profiles of persons who die by suicide (Linehan, 1986; Murphy, 1986). It is fair to conclude that prior studies provide
some basis for characterizing persons likely to make nonfatal
suicide attempts, persons likely to make serious nonfatal
attempts, and persons likely to repeat nonfatal attempt behavior—but that knowledge about those who actually kill
themselves is much less adequate.

Of course, the process is a mutual one, as clinical understanding influences epidemiologic knowledge. For instance, clinicians reporting on individual cases or small
numbers of cases may explore in depth such issues as the
character structure of the suicidal or homicidal adolescent,
the availability of firearms, substance abuse, and so on. Such
information is then picked up and used in larger epidemiologic studies. This pattern of ongoing, mutual exchange of
information between the epidemiologic and clinical perspectives is discussed more fully in Chapter 3.

Epidemiologic studies are also the best platform for studying, planning, and evaluating public health policy interventions. Epidemiologic data can identify risk factors that lie outside the usual scope of psychiatric practice, thus suggesting societal in addition to individual interventions to lower suicide and homicide rates. Public health policies, prevention strategies, and intervention programs should be guided by both epidemiologic and clinical data, but this common-sense approach often seems the exception rather than the rule.

OVERVIEW OF THIS BOOK

There were three reasons for our writing this book. First, as noted above, the similarity of long-term mortality patterns of suicide and homicide among youth suggests that these problems may be related at least epidemiologically and that exploring them together may be useful. Second, also as noted above, we wanted to focus on the potential integration of epidemiologic and clinical frames of reference in the areas of youth suicide and homicide. Third, a fresh look at this problem should allow us to update various aspects of the data.

In Chapter 2, the problem of suicide and homicide among youth is introduced. Suicide and homicide deaths among adolescents are discussed in the context of other forms of mortality, and patterns in the literature are presented.

In Chapter 3, the theoretical concerns raised above are discussed at greater length. How can the epidemiologic as well as the clinical perspective enhance an understanding of youth suicide and homicide? What are the relationships between the clinical and epidemiologic viewpoints? How does one understand the relationships between suicide and homicide?

In Chapters 4 through 6, three aspects of the problem are discussed: (1) the epidemiology of suicide and homicide among the young in the United States (Chapter 4); (2) the potential for demographic and economic variables to enhance our understanding of suicide and homicide among youth, and possibly to enable us to predict longitudinal trends (Chapter 5); and (3) the epidemiology of suicide and homicide among youth of other countries (Chapter 6). Various questions are generated in addressing these three issues. For example, Chapter 4 asks: Which age, race, and sex groups are at highest risk of dying by suicide and homicide in the United States? What are the trends over time for suicide and homicide among youth? How are these patterns similar and dissimilar? What factors appear to influence these trends? Chapter 5 addresses the following: Which variables appear to be most closely related to suicide and homicide patterns among youth? Can demographic and economic variables be used to predict violent death trends in youthful populations? If so, can intervention and prevention strategies be developed to reduce suicide and homicide? Chapter 6 asks: What are the age, race, and sex patterns for suicide and homicide among youth in countries and cultures different from the United States? How do these trends differ from those in the United States? Which countries tend to have the highest suicide and homicide rates among youth, and which the lowest?

In Chapters 7 and 8, various clinical perspectives are addressed: Who attempts and completes suicide? Who are the victims and perpetrators of homicide? What clinical and sociocultural factors predispose youth to suicide and homicide? Prevention and intervention strategies are discussed for youth suicide and homicide. For youth suicide, a number of major reviews from varying perspectives are examined. For youth homicide, various strategies in the areas of primary, secondary, and tertiary prevention are explored.

Chapter 9 is an epilogue that concludes the book. In addition to presenting a summary of major points, this chapter presents a discussion of some key clinical and theoretical issues in suicide and homicide among youth.

CHAPTER TWO

The Nature of the Problem

Chapter 2 introduces the problem of youth suicide and homicide: Suicide and homicide among 15- to 24-year-olds account for over 30% of all deaths in that age group. For youth suicide, there has been an explosion of research over the past 15 years which has greatly enhanced our understanding of this phenomenon; by contrast, much less work has been done on youth homicide. Various risk factors for youth suicide and homicide are outlined.

YOUTH SUICIDE AND HOMICIDE IN CONTEXT

Every year, more than 75% of all deaths among 15- to 24-year-olds are caused by violence (suicide, homicide, and accidents). In 1990, 36,733 individuals aged 15–24 died in the United States; of these, 28,464 died violently. Table 2.1 shows that violent deaths account for far more mortality among youth than any other cause of death, with rates much greater than those for cancer, heart disease, and so on. Violent deaths would seem to be *the* medical problem of adolescents and young adults in the United States. Clinicians and researchers must confront this problem, together with the public health community and society at large.

The data on the relative importance of violent deaths among youth can also be presented in more detail. Table 2.2 shows that motor-vehicle accidents are the leading cause of death among those aged 15–24 (34.3% of all deaths), followed by homicide (20.0%), suicide (13.3%), and all other accidents (9.9%), respectively. These data and rankings have been fairly constant for many years (Holinger, 1987). Suicide

9

TABLE 2.1. Deaths in Adolescence: Mortality Rates and Numbers of Deaths among 15- to 24-Year-Olds, United States, 1990, for Selected Causes

	Number of deaths	Mortality rate (per 100,000 population)	% of total[a]
All causes	36,733	99.2	100.0
Violent deaths (suicide, homicide, accidents)	28,464	77.0	77.5
Malignant neoplasm	1,819	4.9	5.0
Major cardiovascular disease	1,224	3.3	3.3
Symptoms, signs, ill-defined conditions	711	1.9	1.9
Congenital anomalies	491	1.3	1.3
Pneumonia and influenza	231	0.6	0.6
All other causes	3,793	10.2	10.3

Source of data: National Center for Health Statistics, *Advance Report of Final Mortality Statistics, 1990,* Monthly Vital Statistics Report, Vol. 41, No. 7, Suppl. Jan. 7, 1993. DHHS Pub. No. (PHS) 93-1120. Hyattsville, MD: U.S. Public Health Service, 1993.
[a]Percentages for selected causes do not total 100% because of rounding.

and homicide can each be seen to account for more deaths among youth than any other single cause, with the exception of accidents. More than 30% of all deaths among 15- to 24-year-olds are caused by suicide and homicide.

In attempting to understand the phenomena of suicide and homicide among adolescents, we should also examine

TABLE 2.2. Violent Deaths in Adolescence: Mortality Rates and Numbers of Deaths among 15- to 24-Year-Olds, United States, 1990

	Number of deaths	Mortality rate (per 100,000 population)[a]	% of total
All causes	36,733	99.2	100.0
Motor-vehicle accidents	12,607	34.1	34.3
Homicide	7,354	19.9	20.0
Suicide	4,869	13.2	13.3
All other accidents	3,634	9.8	9.9
All other causes	8,269	22.3	22.5

Source of data: See Table 2.1.
[a]Rates for selected causes do not total 99.2 because of rounding.

the larger scope of data on violent deaths. In the United States, suicide, homicide, and accidents are the leading causes of death for ages 1–39—more than half of the expected life span (Institute of Medicine, National Academy of Sciences, 1985a; Holinger, 1980). One measure utilized to examine the impact of various causes of mortality is called "years of potential life lost" (Lalonde, 1974). Calculations can be made of the years of potential life lost as a result of each cause, and measured against a life expectancy of, for example, 72 years for men and 76 years for women. More years of expected life are lost because of violent deaths than any other cause, including heart disease and cancer (Institute of Medicine, 1985a; Holinger, 1980). This high proportion of loss can be attributed primarily to suicides, homicides, and accidental deaths among young people. It is also of interest to examine the age patterns for the various causes of violent death. For example, suicide rates tend to increase with age. With the exception of children, adolescents have the lowest suicide rates of any age group. Similarly, non-motor-vehicle accidents tend to be lower for adolescents than for other groups, whereas homicide and motor-vehicle accident rates among the young are higher than for many other age groups.

Cross-cultural comparisons are also of interest. In Chapter 6, Table 6.1 demonstrates that the overall total suicide rate in the United States falls approximately in the bottom third of rates for the various countries studied. In addition, Table 6.1 shows that nearly all countries have age patterns similar to those of the United States—that is, low rates of suicide among youth and an increase in rates with age. Thus, one finds something of a paradox: Adolescent suicide appears to get relatively more attention than does suicide in other age groups; yet cross-cultural data consistently demonstrate that adolescents have lower rates than do other age groups. For homicide, the comparisons with other countries show dramatically different results (see Table 6.2): The homicide rates for the United States are far higher than for nearly any other country (Fingerhut and Kleinman, 1990). In addition, in contrast to the low suicide rates in the 15–24 age group compared with those for adults, homicide rates for 15- to 24-year-olds in the United States are among the highest of any age group in this country. Furthermore, homicide rates for the 15–24 age group in the United States are higher than those for 15- to 24-year-olds in nearly every other country studied: The rates are five times higher than those for any country other than Mexico (see Table 6.2; Fingerhut and Kleinman, 1990).

There is increasing evidence to suggest that the trends of violent deaths are not random, but are understandable from both clinical and epidemiologic perspectives. This notion may give us some hope of effectively intervening and perhaps preventing at least some of this loss of life and potential.

The scientific exploration of violent deaths among the young is itself a relatively new endeavor. The first major comprehensive literature review of adolescent suicide was conducted by Seiden in 1969, and he found approximately 200 publications on the topic. Since then, however, there has been a dramatic increase in the number of articles and books in this area. Work by investigators such as Sudak et al. (1984), Rosenberg et al. (1987), Pfeffer (1989), Griffith and Bell (1989), and Fingerhut and Kleinman (1990), as well as the *Report of the Secretary's Task Force on Youth Suicide* (1989), has greatly enhanced our understanding of violent deaths among youth. The psychodynamic and clinical aspects, cluster phenomena, biologic factors, and epidemiologic patterns are now much more closely studied than they were a few years ago.

The systematic scientific study of adolescence is particularly important, given the curiously contradictory impressions of adolescent mental health. On the one hand, adolescents are often seen as being in turmoil, and the attention given by the mass media to suicide among adolescents seems to convey the idea that rates among this age group are far higher than rates for other ages. On the other hand, with long lives in front of them, adolescents are often seen as having little "reason" to kill themselves (unlike older persons, for whom suicide seems more "understandable"). Newspaper reports following an adolescent suicide frequently initially portray the youth as an "All-American kid" with no problems, and family and friends as completely shocked at the event. Thus, the tendency exists to generalize adolescent mental health as being excessively good or excessively poor (Offer and Schonert-Reichl, 1992). However, epidemiologic studies indicate that the prevalence of psychiatric disorder among adolescents is about 15%–20% (Offer and Sabshin, 1984a)—that is, almost identical to the prevalence rates found among adults (Klerman and Weissman, 1984). Furthermore, contrary to the impression given by the media attention to youth suicide, the suicide rates among adolescents are consistently *lower* than for adult age groups (Kramer et al., 1972; Holinger, 1987). Therefore, the increased scientific study of adolescent mental health and mortality is a welcome advance.

Despite this increase in our understanding of youthful violent mortality, however, age, period, and cohort variables still appear to be the major factors in the increases and decreases of violent mortality time trends among youth. The disquieting question remains: Can explicit interventions generated from this new knowledge result in any consistent decrease in the rate of violent mortality among youth?

The focus of this book, as its title indicates, is on suicide and homicide among youth. Suicide is a reflection of overt self-destructiveness, and homicide may reflect a more subtle form of self-destructive behavior. Homicide rates refer specifically to those who are killed, and say nothing about the killers. Wolfgang (1959), who studied several hundred homicides in detail, found that more than 25% were overtly provoked by the victim. He suggested that these deaths were "suicide by means of victim-precipitated homicide" (Wolfgang, 1959). Interestingly, the longitudinal epidemiologic patterns of suicide and homicide are quite similar (see Chapter 3). There is an extensive literature on the similarities and dissimilarities between suicide and homicide, and these issues are discussed in more detail below. Accident mortality has also been conceptualized in terms of self-destructive tendencies (risk-taking behaviors and "accident-proneness"), but the data relative to accident mortality and self-destructiveness are conflicting; in addition, the longitudinal epidemiologic data on accidents are less clearly related to suicide than are the homicide data (Holinger, 1987). Thus, it seems to serve conceptual clarity to detail the relationships between suicide and homicide data in the present work.

PATTERNS IN THE LITERATURE

Comprehensive literature reviews and updates have been presented elsewhere (e.g., Pfeffer, 1989; *Report of the Secretary's Task Force on Youth Suicide,* 1989; Sudak et al., 1984; Holinger and Offer, 1981; Rosenberg et al., 1987; Griffith and Bell, 1989; Fingerhut and Kleinman, 1990); rather than repeat their findings in detail here, we address the various patterns in the literature. The literature dealing with data, etiology, treatment, and prevention is discussed in greater detail in later chapters.

Suicide

The past decade has seen the emergence of a new scientific field within suicidology—one dealing specifically with suicide among the young. In describing the development of recent work in self-destructive tendencies among the young, we need to put the problem into perspective. As stated above, in the first major literature review, Seiden (1969) noted that approximately 200 articles and books were available on the topic at that time; he provided the field with a comprehensive analysis of various aspects of adolescent suicide. Another literature review approximately 10 years later (Holinger and Offer, 1981) noted that since Seiden's review the number of publications had approximately doubled. Just 3 years later, Sudak et al. (1984) presented a series of research papers that conveyed not only an explosion of data and publications on youthful suicide, but also the establishment of viable, growing subsections within that field. Further evidence of the emergence of youthful suicide as a specific field of scientific inquiry is seen in two recent publications: the U.S. Department of Health and Human Services' *Report of the Secretary's Task Force on Youth Suicide* (1989), and the American Psychiatric Press's *Suicide among Youth: Perspectives on Risk and Prevention* (Pfeffer, 1989).

Interestingly, this increase in the scientific literature on youth suicide has corresponded to a steady increase in adolescent suicide rates. In the mid-1950s, the suicide rates for young people were at the lowest points recorded in this century in the United States. Then the rates began increasing to their highest recorded rates in the late 1970s, with a subsequent tendency toward leveling off (see Chapter 3).

Various perspectives in studying adolescent suicide have been advanced in the literature; until recently, one could categorize them more or less coherently as biologic, psychologic, and social perspectives. Recent studies, however, have begun to create intricate bridges between individual and group dynamics, which enhance our knowledge but defy easy categorization. This research involves epidemiologic patterns as well as demographic and economic variables.

In the clinical research, the summaries of youth suicide patterns from previous decades (Seiden, 1969; Holinger and Offer, 1981) have gradually been enhanced by increasingly sophisticated studies performed more recently (*Report of the Secretary's Task Force on Youth Suicide*, 1989; Sudak et al., 1984; Pfeffer, 1989; Blumenthal and Kupfer, 1988; Rosenberg et al., 1987; Klerman et al., 1985), as noted above. From these and other investigations, we attempt to glean major risk factors and attributes.

The literature indicates that white males are at greatest risk in the 15–19 and 20–24 age groups. Several risk factors emerge to aid in identifying those youth at highest risk. First, both retrospective and prospective research suggests that most youth who kill themselves meet the criteria for diagnosable psychiatric disorders (Fowler et al., 1986; Rich et al., 1986; Runesen, 1989; Blumenthal and Kupfer, 1988; Shafii et al., 1985; Shaffer et al., 1985; Brent et al., 1988). Affective disorders (either bipolar disorder or major depression) have been found in approximately 25%–75% of youthful suicides (Runesen, 1989; Brent et al., 1988; Shafii, 1986; Rich et al., 1986), and personality disorders (especially borderline) have been found in 25%–40% (Shaffer et al., 1985; Runesen, 1989; Rich et al., 1986; Blumenthal and Kupfer, 1988). Second, studies indicate that approximately 25%–50% of youth who kill themselves have a family history of psychiatric disorder and/or suicide (Roy, 1989; Blumenthal and Kupfer, 1988; Brent et al., 1988; Shafii et al., 1985). Third, approximately 25%–50% of youth who complete suicide have made previous suicide attempts, with the number of attempts and lethality of attempts being positively correlated with ultimate suicide (Farberow, 1989; Shafii et al., 1985; Brent et al., 1988; Blumenthal and Kupfer, 1988). Fourth, high percentages (33%–70%) of youthful suicides have abused alcohol or drugs (Runesen, 1989; Shafii et al., 1985; Rich et al., 1986; Fowler et al., 1986; Schuckit and Schuckit, 1989). Comorbidity of affective disorders, personality disorders, and/or substance abuse appears to be particularly lethal (Blumenthal and Kupfer, 1988; Brent et al., 1988; Shafii et al., 1988). Fifth, the proportion of firearms accounting for adolescent suicide has increased recently (Mościcki and Boyd, 1983–1985), and firearms in the homes of suicidal or potentially suicidal adolescents have been shown to markedly increase their risk for suicide (Brent et al., 1991; Rosenberg et al., 1991). Sixth, gender identity issues, including homosexuality, also appear to represent a risk factor for youth suicide (Remafedi et al., 1991; Judson, 1993).

Clinical studies of suicide among youth, such as those from which the risk factors described above are derived, have reached a very high level of sophistication over the past decade. However, they are not without their methodologic problems (Lann et al., 1989), two of which should be noted here. First, most such studies consist of data from psychologic autopsies and are retrospective rather than prospective. These studies are subject to limitation of amount of data, as well as various biases (Lann et al., 1989). Second, the control groups used have consisted of psychiatric inpatients, suicidal youth, or suicides from older age groups; there is a lack of research using youth in the general population as controls. Hence, it is difficult to determine the importance of the above-described risk factors and their relative risk values in the context of the general youthful population.

Much research has been conducted recently on biologic aspects of depression and suicide, but this work has tended to involve adult rather than adolescent populations. Ambrosini et al. (1984) and Goodwin and Brown (1989) have reviewed this literature and suggested that some evidence exists for specific biologic factors underlying some adolescent depressions and suicides. It appears well documented that major affective disorders (major depression and bipolar disorder) and schizophrenia have a genetic component; these disorders are seen in adolescence and are associated with rates of suicide far higher than seen in the general population.

To turn to psychodynamic factors, both dyadic and triadic issues are seen in suicidal adolescents (Anthony, 1970). Recently, Hendin (1991a) has ably reviewed many of the psychodynamic issues involved in youth suicide: rage; hopelessness, despair, desperation; guilt; rebirth and reunion; retaliatory abandonment; revenge; and self-punishment and atonement. Haim's (1974) detailed study focused on suicidal adolescents' inability to disinvest the disappointing or lost object. Extensive clinical data have highlighted major dynamic themes, such as identification with lost objects, the role of hostility from significant others, and countertransference issues (Cain, 1972; Sabbath, 1969; Rosenbaum and Richman, 1970; Hurry, 1977, 1978; Kernberg, 1974; Laufer, 1974; Novick, 1984; Maltsberger and Buie, 1974). In addition, patients with self disorders, self-esteem pathology, vulnerability to fragmentation, and vulnerability to suicide (i.e., those with borderline and narcissistic personality disorders) have been increasingly described by theorists in object relations and self psychology (Kernberg, 1975; Kohut, 1971, 1984; Reiser, 1986; Kavka, 1976).

The possibility that suicide clusters or contagion may represent another risk factor for adolescent suicide has been the focus of a variety of studies over the past decade. A "suicide cluster" may be defined as a group of suicide attempts that occur closer together in time and space than would normally be expected in a given community (Centers for Disease Control [CDC], 1988a). Statistical analysis of national mortality data has suggested that clusters of completed suicide occur predominantly among adolescents and young adults, and that such clusters may account for approximately 1%–5% of all suicides in this age group (Gould et al., 1987). Much anecdotal evidence suggests that suicide clusters may occur through "contagion"; that is, suicides occurring later in a cluster often appear to have been influenced by suicides occurring earlier in the cluster through mechanisms of identification and imitation (Davidson and Gould, 1989). However, detailed studies supporting this hypothesis are not yet available (Davidson and Gould, 1989), and one recent study specifically did *not* demonstrate increased exposure to media presentations of suicide among teenagers who killed themselves (Davidson and Gould, 1989). Detailed research, however, has been conducted on two other aspects of suicide contagion: fictionalized TV portrayals of suicide (serials and movies), and media news reports of actual suicide. Studies of fictional portrayals of suicide on TV have found data both supporting (e.g., Gould and Shaffer, 1986; Phillips, 1982) and contradicting (e.g., Berman, 1988; Phillips and Paight, 1987; Kessler and Stipp, 1984) the hypothesis that such TV shows are related to an increase in suicide. Similarly, some research supports a relationship between media news reports (TV and newspapers) of actual suicide and an increase in suicide rates (e.g., Phillips and Carstensen, 1986; Phillips, 1979), while other work does not support the hypothesis (e.g., Kessler et al., 1988; Baron and Reiss, 1985). The relationship, then, between media accounts of suicide (both fictionalized and nonfictionalized) and shifts in teenage suicide rates is at present extremely scientifically controversial (Davidson and Gould, 1989). Thus, perhaps the most we can say, given the current data, is that some evidence suggests that exposing the youthful population to suicide through the mass media may increase the risk of suicide for certain susceptible individuals (CDC, 1988a).

Sociocultural investigations have focused on economic and demographic variables, and these are described in more detail later. It should be noted here, however, that several studies (including cohort analyses and cross-cultural work) have documented the increase in adolescent suicide and depression over the years from the mid-1950s to the early 1980s (Murphy and Wetzel, 1980; Solomon and Hellon, 1980; Klerman et al., 1985). In addition, evidence suggests that demographic variables (the increased proportion of adolescents) and economic variables (increased unemployment) were related to the increases in adolescent suicide rates (Easterlin, 1980; Brenner, 1971, 1979; Holinger and Offer, 1981, 1982; Holinger et al., 1987; Hendin, 1982).

Homicide

Scientific studies of homicide among youth have lagged even behind those for youth suicide. This research is described in more detail in Chapter 8, but some basic issues should be noted here. Christoffel (1990) has suggested that childhood homicides are of two types: (1) infantile (i.e., fatal injury of infants up to 1 year of age by caretakers), the overwhelming pattern in very early childhood; and (2) adolescent (i.e., fatal injury in the community), the dominant pattern in preadolescence and beyond. This study supports others showing that 5- to 9-year-olds are at least risk of dying by homicide (Holinger et al., 1983–1985). In the infantile pattern, death is most often attributable to beatings. In the adolescent pattern, death can be attributed to firearms, hit-and-run crashes, strangulations, and so on. Deaths caused by firearms increase with age from early adolescence (10–14 years) to middle–late adolescence (15–19 years) to young adulthood (20–24 years). High firearm injury rates are associated with poverty, minority status, population density, prevalence of guns in the community, and proximity of available gun purchase (Christoffel, 1990).

Victims and perpetrators of youth homicide share a number of characteristics. Older African-American adolescents are at greatest risk of becoming homicide victims. However, the specific age, sex, race, and other characteristics of the victim appear closely related to the type of homicide committed (i.e., assault homicide, robbery homicide, burglary homicide, or rape homicide) (Block, 1986). The bulk of the evidence suggests that most homicide victims know their killers (Block, 1986; Miller, 1983; Christoffel, 1990). Fingerhut and Kleinman (1990) noted that for 1987, of the 72% of homicides among males aged 15–24 years with known victims and offenders, 90% of African-American male victims were murdered by African-American persons and 87% of white male victims were murdered by white persons. Furthermore, 68% of white and 76% of African-American male victims were murdered by someone who was known to them (Fingerhut and Kleinman, 1990).

The risk of becoming a homicide victim appears to be closely related to poverty and urban dwelling (Christoffel, 1990; Muscat, 1988; Ropp, et al., 1992; Flango and Sherbonou, 1976; Williams, 1984; Loftin and Hill, 1974). Some studies suggest that the poverty variable is so strong that when socioeconomic status is controlled for, the racial differences in homicide rates decrease substantially (Williams, 1984; Christoffel, 1990; Griffith and Bell, 1989; CDC, 1986, 1988b; Tardiff, 1987). Alcohol and other drugs also appear to be related to the risk of becoming a homicide victim (Griffith and Bell, 1989). Studies of large samples of homicide victims aged 15–24 have shown that many (approximately 20%–40%) were legally intoxicated or had alcohol in their blood (Goodman et al., 1986; Christoffel, 1990). Another study found that nearly half of over 200 homicide victims had significant blood levels of cocaine's major metabolite, benzoylecgonine (Hanzlick and Gowitt, 1991). Finally, there is a dearth of studies dealing with the psychological character structure of homicide victims. However, several researchers have suggested that a large percentage of homicides are victim-precipitated—in other words, that the victims provoke their own deaths to some extent (e.g., Wolfgang, 1968; MacDonald, 1961).

With respect to the perpetrators of homicide among

adolescents, data suggest that homicide offenders tend to match victims on race and age (Christoffel, 1990; Block, 1986). Teen/youth gang involvement has been implicated in about 25% of teen murders (Christoffel, 1990), and one study found that more than 50% of homicides attributed to teens are committed by multiple offenders—that is, gangs (Block, 1986). This tendency to commit murder in a group was found to decline rapidly with age (Block, 1986). Federal Bureau of Investigation data indicate that for African-American homicide victims aged 15–24 who died between 1976 and 1984, almost two-thirds were killed during an argument or other nonfelony, and more than half of the victims were killed by persons known to them (mostly non-relatives) (O'Carroll, 1988). Homicide offenders aged 18–34 have been found to be more likely than controls to have been in juvenile detention, and more likely to have low education levels and to carry guns; victims of nonfatal gun or knife assault had the same risk factors, except that they were less likely than offenders to carry guns (Christoffel, 1990).

Relationships between Suicide and Homicide

Henry and Short (1954), in their early epidemiologic studies of specific localities over time spans of a few years, suggested that suicide and homicide were inversely related. More recently, longitudinal studies of suicide and homicide rates for the entire United States over several decades have suggested a different pattern—namely, that suicide and homicide rates among the young are strikingly *parallel* over time (e.g., Klebba, 1975; Holinger and Klemen, 1982; Holinger et al., 1987). Brenner's (1971, 1979) and Easterlin's (1980) work on economic and demographic variables, respectively, implies that suicide and homicide rates increase and decrease during roughly the same time periods.

To turn to the epidemiologic patterns of murder-suicide, studies show that the incidence of this combination for various countries is remarkably constant, averaging about 0.20–0.30 per 100,000 population (Marzuk et al., 1992a). In the United States, murder–suicide accounts for about 1.5% of all suicides and 5% of all homicides annually (Marzuk et al., 1992). Some researchers have suggested that the higher the rate of homicide in a population, the lower the percentage of murder–suicide. Thus, although the proportion of murder–suicide among all homicides is as low as 5% in a country with a high homicide rate such as the United States, it ranges as high as 22% in Australia, 33% in England, and 42% in Denmark, countries with lower homicide rates (Rosenbaum, 1990; Clark, 1990; Marzuk et al., 1992).

Clinically, the literature on murder–suicides indicates that most (one-half to three-fourths) occur in the home after the female victims have spurned (or are perceived to have spurned) the male perpetrators (Clark, 1990; Rosenbaum, 1990). Studies of large samples of murdered children aged 16 years and younger have consistently shown that the perpetrators are biological or foster parents in 54%–78% of all cases. It is estimated that 20%–22% of the perpetrators die by suicide and that an additional 4%–17% subsequently make nonfatal suicide attempts. In general, it has been found that suicidal men with diagnosable depressions sometimes kill their wives and children before making an attempt on their own lives; suicidal women with diagnosable depressions are less likely to kill their husbands, but sometimes kill their children before making an attempt on their own lives (Clark, 1990; Rosenbaum, 1990).

CHAPTER THREE

A Theoretical Framework

Chapter 3 discusses theoretical issues. It is suggested that utilizing both epidemiologic and clinical perspectives is essential to gaining a more complete understanding of youth suicide and homicide. In addition, various levels of abstraction and interaction between the epidemiologic and clinical arenas are presented.

In any attempt at a better understanding of youth suicide and homicide, at least two theoretical tasks are necessary, as we have noted briefly in Chapter 1. The first of these is integrating epidemiologic and clinical perspectives; the second is exploring the relationships between suicide and homicide. We are aware that both of these are difficult tasks; however, if the attempt sheds some new light on the problem of youth suicide and homicide, it will have been worth the effort.

INTEGRATION OF EPIDEMIOLOGIC AND CLINICAL PERSPECTIVES

External Stress and Internal Vulnerability

The difficulty of the youth suicide and homicide problem suggests that as complete a picture as possible be used to try to understand it. There are tremendous amounts of epidemiologic data and clinical data dealing with youth suicide and homicide. Yet usually this problem is addressed from only one narrow aspect or another. It would seem that a broader approach is necessary—one that pulls together various patterns in the data. Only then, it would seem, can truly logical and coherent intervention and prevention strategies be devised.

How do epidemiologic and clinical perspectives relate? "Epidemiology" refers to the frequency and distribution of disease (MacMahon and Pugh, 1970). The term "clinical" involves the symptoms and course of the disease of individual patients (*Stedman's Medical Dictionary*, 1966). Epidemiology, then, relates in a sense to the external patterns and pressures involved in a disease process, whereas the clinical perspective tends to focus more on internal factors. To put it differently, epidemiology refers more to external pressures or risk factors; the clinical viewpoint refers more to the internal vulnerabilities. Needless to say, there is certainly overlap between these external and internal perspectives. It is not always clear what external "reality" is, or how that may be mediated internally. Philosophers and psychologists have wrestled for centuries with the question of what is outside, what is inside, and how one articulates the difference (e.g., Goldberg, 1990). And yet, despite the overlapping and the difficulty in conceptualizing the problem, it seems that our attempt to achieve a better understanding of youth suicide and homicide depends on a consideration of both perspectives.

Most illnesses can benefit from an exploration of both external risk factors and internal vulnerabilities. For example, most of us are exposed constantly to various bacteria that can cause pneumonia; yet we usually only get sick with pneumonia if we are debilitated in some way (i.e., if we manifest an internal vulnerability together with the external agent). Cardiac mortality may be viewed similarly: Internal factors (e.g., heredity, type of lipoprotein, how one's body handles cholesterol, etc.) can tip the scales for or against a heart attack, but when certain external stresses (e.g., loss of job, death in the family, sustained exertion in cold weather) are added to increased internal vulnerability, the risk of heart attack in an individual becomes quite high. The issue of the overlapping of the external and internal viewpoints is apparent in this example, as intriguing questions arise regarding how such factors as loss of job or death in the family are mediated internally to increase the risk of a heart attack. On a more macroscopic level, Brenner's work is of interest (Brenner, 1971, 1979); he found positive correlations between periods of unemployment and cardiac mortality over time for large geographic areas. A third example can be taken from psychiatry. Schizophrenia appears to be an illness that involves an internal vulnerability (an inherited biochemical or structural predisposition to developing the episodes of delusions and hallucinations characteristic of schizophrenia) combined with external (environmental) stresses. Support for this idea comes from studies of schizophrenic parents of identical twins who were separated at birth. A twin raised by the schizophrenic parents had more chance of developing schizophrenia than a twin raised by nonschizophrenic parents, but both twins had a greater chance of developing schizophrenia than was found in the general population.

Microscopic and Macroscopic: Different Levels of Abstraction

What also emerges in attempting to integrate epidemiologic and clinical perspectives is that this needs to be done on different levels of abstraction. At least two levels of possible integration exist: the microscopic (dealing more with individual cases) and the macroscopic (involving entire populations and issues of services, policy, etc.).

The Microscopic Level

On the microscopic level, an understanding of epidemiologic data can be used to aid in the assessment and treatment of individual cases in the clinical situation. For example, suppose an elderly white man comes into the emergency room complaining of various somatic problems, sleeplessness, and depression. The intake worker learns that he is a widower (his wife died 1½ years ago), lives alone, and is no longer working. These data can be used to alert the physician and staff about possible suicide risk in this patient; the patient's being male, white, elderly, widowed, unemployed, and living alone are important epidemiologic risk factors for suicide. Of course, a complete physical and psychiatric evaluation of the patient's depression and other symptoms will be necessary for an adequate assessment of whether or not this man is actually suicidal. Yet it is precisely this group (elderly white men living alone, etc.) that has the highest suicide rate in the United States, and an understanding of the significance of these epidemiologic risk factors can be a very valuable aid in the clinical assessment of such patients.

As another example, suppose that a 17-year-old African-American girl is brought to the emergency room by her mother, who tells the physician that over the past 2 days her daughter has been increasingly jittery and complaining of wanting to crawl out of her skin. The physician learns that the girl has a 3-year history of schizophrenia, and that the illness has been in remission for the past year; in addition, the doctor discovers that the girl's father, a successful attorney, is an avid hunter and keeps several guns in the house. Here the contribution of the epidemiologic data is a bit more complex. On the one hand, young nonwhite women have the lowest suicide rates in this country; on the other hand, the girl's history of schizophrenia and the availability of guns in the house greatly increase the suicide risk.

Clinical cases and data on the microscopic level can also influence epidemiologic work. Clinicians begin reporting about and describing their individual cases or small groups of cases, and certain patterns begin to emerge with respect to location, numbers, and attributes of the patients. For example, clinical reports during the early 1980s began to relate youth suicide to substance abuse and availability of firearms in the home (*Report of the Secretary's Task Force on Youth Suicide*, 1989). Recently a series of epidemiologic studies, using case–control formats and examining large numbers of youth suicides, added two more important pieces of information to the current understanding of youth suicide (Brent et al., 1991). First, substance abuse and the character pathology underlying it were found to be important risk factors; furthermore, substance abuse in a youngster with a major psychiatric disorder (major depression, bipolar disorder, or schizophrenia) was shown to be a particularly lethal combination. Second, the presence of a gun in the home of a youngster was found to be a significant risk factor for youth suicide. These epidemiologic findings and generalizations, then, originated in observations on the clinical level.

Of course, the process does not stop there. As these important epidemiologic findings on substance abuse and firearm availability become increasingly widespread, various clinicians from psychiatrists to social workers to emergency room personnel will (let us hope) use them to enhance their assessment of potentially suicidal youth. For example, it now appears difficult to overestimate the importance of actively intervening on a clinical basis with the bipolar youngster who shows signs of substance abuse, or with the gun-owning family that has a depressed teen at home. Thus, characteristically in psychiatry as well as other medical fields, there appears to exist an interaction between the epidemiologic and clinical areas. The specific clinical cases generate ideas and hypotheses, which are then explored on the large epidemiologic level, and these generalizations in turn ultimately influence clinical practice. There is, then, a constant interchange of information between the epidemiologic and clinical perspectives.

The Macroscopic Level

On the macroscopic level, at issue is the interaction of the epidemiologic and clinical viewpoints at the level of entire populations. Epidemiologic information is critical in terms of informing the decisions made with respect to resources in clinical medicine. Issues such as types of physician training programs, clinical services, medical technology, and the like are all dependent on epidemiologic data. For example, funding decisions regarding suicide and homicide are based on determining what populations are at risk and addressing the various treatment, prevention, and research issues. This is the task of epidemiology, and this endeavor has a profound effect on the health of the populations involved. Again, there is an interaction between the epidemiologic and clinical perspectives. As various programs are put into effect to enhance the health of a particular population, there is constant feedback regarding the clinical status of the members of that population. This clinical feedback, in turn, provides information on the epidemiologic level regarding the efficacy of such interventions.

Etiology, Assessment/Treatment, and Prevention

It has been suggested that, despite flaws and overlapping, the epidemiologic and clinical perspectives on youth suicide and homicide can be usefully integrated in terms of external stresses and internal vulnerabilities. This integration can now be used to explore various aspects of the etiology, assessment/treatment, and prevention of youth suicide and homicide. A few examples of the epidemiologic–clinical interaction in these contexts are discussed here; more detailed descriptions are presented throughout the rest of the book.

Etiology

With respect to youth suicide, epidemiology can greatly enhance an understanding of causality. Adolescents who are older, white, and male are at greater risk than their counterparts; gun and drug availability increases the risk further, as possibly do increases in the cohort size of adolescents and in unemployment. The major clinical factor, or area of internal vulnerability, that increases the risk of adolescent suicide is the presence of a major psychiatric disorder such as bipolar illness, major depression, or schizophrenia; other clinical risk factors include a positive family history (e.g., for suicide or psychiatric illness) and character structure (especially borderline) of the adolescent.

In terms of youth homicide, the epidemiologic risk factors for both victim and perpetrator include age (older), race (nonwhite), sex (male), poverty, family violence, gun and drug availability, and gang involvement. By contrast, the clinical perspective currently contributes much less to an understanding of either victims or perpetrators of youth homicide. Impulsivity, substance abuse, and those aspects of character structure that lead to gang involvement are apparently risk factors for both victims and perpetrators of youth homicide. It is also possible that the character structure of victims is marked by self-destructive tendencies, whereas the character structure of perpetrators involves aspects of paranoia and projection. However, clinical contributions to the etiology of youth homicide are very scanty, and much more research is necessary in the area.

Assessment and Treatment

Although the assessment and treatment of suicidal youth are primarily clinical endeavors, a knowledge of epidemiologic data can aid in this process. For example, some appreciation of the various high-risk external factors mentioned above in the discussion of etiology can aid the triage emergency room nurse, teachers, and parents, as well as the clinician, in the assessment and treatment of a potentially suicidal youngster. An epidemiologic–clinical integration, combining these epidemiologic data with the relevant clinical information described above and the youngster's current state, would appear to be the most effective way to assess and treat a suicidal youth.

With respect to youth homicide, an epidemiologic–clinical integration seems especially critical, inasmuch as there is such a paucity of clinical data on the assessment and treatment of victims and perpetrators. Most of the current assessment and treatment programs (see Chapter 8) operate on the macroscopic level and use the epidemiologic data mentioned above (poverty, family violence, etc.). This information is essential to politicians and social planners, as well as to teachers, parents, police officers, and others who may deal more with individuals. As noted above, there appear to be few clinical data on the victims and perpetrators of most current youth homicides. However, some clinical information about victims (e.g., the person who disavows knowledge of dangerous circumstances and consistently ends up in "the wrong place at the wrong time") and perpetrators (e.g., the psychotic, paranoid killer) is well known and is being used by clinicians for assessment and treatment.

Prevention

Many of the prevention issues have been raised above in the discussion of assessment and treatment, but prevention tends to have a more macroscopic, epidemiologic focus, as contrasted with the more microscopic clinical aspects of assessment and treatment.

Again, unemployment, gun and medication availability, drugs, and large adolescent cohorts are all epidemiologic variables that have been at least tentatively associated with increased rates of youth suicide. For each of these variables, various researchers and governmental agencies can develop strategies to lessen the impact of these variables; ideally, a decrease in youth suicide should result (if the associations have an etiologic basis) (see Chapter 7). In addition, epidemiologic and clinical issues are combined in prevention strategies involving the training of professionals and paraprofessionals in recognizing potentially suicidal youth. Improved, large-scale suicide assessment training of health workers, clergy, teachers, and others might have a very real effect on the clinical course of the individual lives of troubled youth, and hence on epidemiologic rates as well. Similarly, public education for parents and adolescents on the signs, symptoms, and treatment of youth suicide could have an impact on both the clinical and epidemiologic levels.

With respect to youth homicide, unemployment, poverty, gun availability, drugs, domestic violence, and gang involvement are some of the associated epidemiologic variables that have been the target of preventive strategies. Various social programs are being devised to deal not only with the social conditions that appear to contribute to youth homicide, but also the psychologic issues (e.g., the frustration, hopelessness, rage, paranoia, traumatic reactions, etc.) involved clinically. Public education and training are critical here, both in alerting government and social planners to the epidemiologic variables and in enhancing the capacity of police and health workers to deal with the clinical manifestations.

EXPLORATION OF RELATIONSHIPS BETWEEN SUICIDE AND HOMICIDE

The second theoretical issue dealt with throughout this book is that of exploring the relationships between suicide and homicide. Although the bulk of the book is geared to addressing various aspects of these relationships, a brief description of them may be useful at this point.

Suicide and homicide among youth appear linked in at least two important ways: epidemiologically and psychodynamically. With respect to epidemiology, the suicide and homicide rates for youth are dramatically similar (see Figures 4.9 and 4.10). Not only are the numbers themselves comparable (with homicide rates tending to be slightly higher), but the period effects over the past six decades are quite similar (high rates during the 1930s, lower rates in the 1940s and 1950s, increases throughout the 1960s and 1970s, and some recent leveling off). In addition, evidence appears to suggest that youth suicide and homicide respond to similar social pressures on an epidemiologic level. War, the economy, population shifts, and the availability of guns and drugs seem to have similar associations with suicide and homicide rates. For instance, rates decrease during declared wars (such as World War II) and increase during other periods. Unemployment is also associated with higher suicide and homicide rates, and lower rates are associated with a better economy; this phenomenon may be attributable to the losses of services and training programs providing assessment and treatment for potential suicide and homicide victims and perpetrators, as well as to the direct psychologic effects of economic disaster on individuals. Moreover, large youthful cohorts are associated with higher suicide and homicide rates, and smaller cohorts with lower rates—a pattern that may be attributable to the psychologic and economic deprivations from which the large cohorts suffer. These various epidemiologic relationships between youth suicide and homicide are discussed in greater detail throughout the book.

To turn to psychodynamic links, Sigmund Freud was one of the first to explore the relationships between suicide and homicide (Freud, 1917/1957). The focus has been primarily on the issue of aggression. The dynamics of suicide include the formulation that at least some suicides result from inwardly directed aggression—rage at the self, at an aspect of the self, and/or at an internalized object from the past. Perpetrators of homicide are seen as directing the aggression externally—toward objects in the outside world, with the paranoia, rage, projection, and so forth that accompany this process. Homicide rates, however, actually refer to homicide victims, (i.e., those killed). These victims may include those who both put themselves into potentially dangerous situations (inwardly directed aggression) and also exhibit outwardly directed aggression similar to that manifested by homicide perpetrators in gang activity.

In addition to aggression, dyadic and narcissistic issues also appear to play a role in both youth suicide and homicide. For potential suicide victims, manifestations of character pathology (tension regulation problems, impulsivity, eating disorders, etc.) are all related to self-esteem and dyadic concerns. Such external issues as a poor economy or a large cohort could have a potentially tragic effect on those vulnerable youth with severe narcissistic pathology: Various psychologic and physical needs will go unattended, and an increase in rates may be the result. Moreover, treatment is potentially compromised in the face of those external hardships because of relatively fewer clinicians, facilities, and training programs. Similarly, dyadic and narcissistic issues are involved in youth homicide. The adolescent's longing to belong and to be admired are critical issues in gang activity, and impulsivity and disregard for self and others are characteristic of both youthful homicide victims and perpetrators.

Various treatment and prevention issues emerge from exploring the psychodynamic relationships between youth suicide and homicide. Perhaps one of the most important is the necessity of conveying on a larger level what is known about infant development, affects, and psychologic necessities for rearing a healthier cohort of children. Some of this education is already being carried out by various school systems in work with both parents and children.

CHAPTER FOUR

Epidemiologic Patterns: United States

In the United States, epidemiologic data for adolescents demonstrate that longitudinal shifts in suicide rates are markedly similar to shifts in homicide rates. Older white adolescent males are at greatest risk of suicide, whereas older African-American adolescent males are at greatest risk of dying by homicide. Various data on time trends, current rates, and methods are presented.

It is difficult to overestimate the importance of studying longitudinal data (i.e., studying patterns of suicide and homicide over long periods of time). Not only can examining long-term trends aid in understanding the reasons for ebbs and flows in suicide and homicide rates, but such evaluation also can help in preventing the short-sighted sensationalism that often pervades work in this area.

The purpose of this chapter, then, is to present recent as well as longitudinal epidemiologic data for suicide and homicide among middle and late adolescents and young adults in the United States. The suicide and homicide rates are presented by age, race, and sex for 15- to 24-year-olds. The focus here is on age and period effects; cohort effects are discussed in greater detail in Chapter 5.

METHODOLOGIC ISSUES

A number of serious methodologic problems emerge when epidemiologic data are used. Several such issues are specific to the data analyses presented in the following chapters and are discussed there. However, many problems are of a more general nature and are described here.

Some basic epidemiologic concepts first require description. The "incidence" of a disease is the number of cases of the disease that come into being during a specified period of time. The "incidence rate" is this number per specified unit of population (MacMahon and Pugh, 1970). These concepts of "incidence" need to be distinguished from the term "prevalence." The "point prevalence" of a disease is the frequency of the disease at a designated point in time. The "point prevalence rate" is the proportion of the population exhibiting the disease at that particular time (MacMahon and Pugh, 1970).

"Age-specific rates" are mortality rates for a certain age group, such as individuals aged 15–19 years or 20–24 years. These are the data that are most often utilized in this book. However, some data are "age-adjusted," which is a method of comparing mortality rates over time (or across cultures) while keeping the age structure of the population constant.

Three concepts particularly useful in longitudinal studies are age, period, and cohort effects. "Age effects" involve changes in age-specific rate of mortality or illness over the life span of the individual (Holford, 1983). "Period effects" refer to changes in rate of mortality or illness during a particular historical period (Holford, 1983). "Cohort effects" are differences in rates of mortality or illness among individuals defined by some shared temporal experience, such as year or decade of birth (Holford, 1983).

National mortality rates (number of deaths per population) constitute the major data source for this study.[1] It should be noted that beginning in 1933, the data include the total U.S. population, not samples; prior to 1933, not all states were included in the national mortality data (an issue discussed more fully below). Since the data are primarily in

1. Readers interested in more detailed descriptions of the history and specifics of collecting and analyzing national mortality data are urged to consult the following: *Classification of Terms* . . . (1944), *Death Rates by Age, Race, and Sex* . . . (1956), Klebba and Dolman (1975), Faust and Dolman (1963, 1964, 1965), Dunn and Shackley (1944), and Klebba (1979).

the form of mortality rates (i.e., number of deaths per population), our discussion of methodologic problems is divided into sections investigating problems with calculating the number of deaths and problems with assessing the population. The specific sources of national mortality data are indicated on the individual figures or tables. It should be mentioned, as we address the major questions raised in this book, that the cutoff dates of the data on the figures and tables occasionally vary. These discrepancies in the cutoff date relate to the final year for which data were available when a particular aspect of the study was being conducted, inasmuch as a consistent attempt was made to keep the data as current as possible. This varying of cutoff dates is distinct from the issue noted above regarding use of data before and after 1933.

Problems with Calculating the Number of Deaths

The major problems in obtaining an accurate count of the number of deaths by suicide and homicide can be divided into two groups: misclassification (errors on the local level) and national changes in classification over time (errors on the national level).

Misclassification

"Misclassification" refers to errors made by physicians, coroners, and the like regarding the cause of death as entered on the death certificate. In other words, misclassification involves problems of data gathering at the most basic, local level—the causes of individual deaths before such data are transmitted to the federal government for national compilations. Difficulties arise because individual coroners and physicians or agencies may have biases or rules that distort the data. For example, a situation existed in one state for some time that a death could be listed as a suicide only if a suicide note were left; hence only the literate could be listed as dying by suicide. Such rules can both decrease numbers and bias the results with respect to age, sex, and racial groups. These kinds of errors in gathering data result in either underreporting or overreporting. Among adolescents, suicide is more likely than homicide to be subject to misclassification errors, and underreporting is the more frequent type of misclassification error for suicide.

Underreporting may be intentional or unintentional. The family or the doctor may intentionally cover up a suicide for a variety of reasons, such as insurance benefits, religious reasons (e.g., for Roman Catholics, suicide may prevent a church funeral and burial), social stigma, guilt, malpractice problems, and so on. Unintentional underreporting may result when actual suicides are classified as accidents simply because there is not enough evidence to support a final determination of suicide. For example, some single-car crashes, overdoses, and poisonings that are actually suicides may be labeled "accidents" because they are unverifiable as suicides. Actual rates of suicide may exceed published rates by a factor of two or three (Seiden, 1969; Toolan, 1962, 1975; Kramer et al., 1972; Holinger, 1990a).

Working with younger age groups poses special problems of misclassification. It may be easier to cover up suicides among the young and call them accidental deaths. Poisoning and other methods of suicide are more easily conceived of as accidents in these age groups than in older age groups. In addition, parents' emotional investment in children and adolescents often creates pressure to make diagnoses other than suicide in younger groups; suicide among the young creates great social stigma and guilt because of such issues as parents' being seen as having been "bad parents." Consistent with these concerns are data from two recent studies: Gist and Welch (1989) and Males (1991) have provided evidence that much of the rise of adolescent suicide from the 1950s through the 1970s may have been artifactual because of misclassification in the past.

National Changes in Classification over Time

The *International List of Diseases and Causes of Death* (also known as the *International Classification of Diseases* or ICD), used in this country since 1900, has been revised about every 10 years so that the disease descriptions will be consistent with advances in medical science and changes in diagnostic practice (Klebba and Dolman, 1975; National Center for Health Statistics, 1980). Each decennial revision has produced some break in the comparability of cause-of-death statistics. For example, say a man tries to kill himself by jumping out a window and survives, but dies 2 weeks later of pneumonia resulting from the internal injuries associated with the fall. One revision of the ICD may classify such a death as a suicide, whereas another may classify it as a result of pneumonia. Overall, the comparability of suicide and homicide data based on the different revisions has been fairly good. Throughout the first four editions of the ICD, suicide and homicide data were comparable; however, quantitative evaluations of the changes created by new editions were not possible. The changes created by the move from the fourth to the fifth edition were quantified as percentages, and the changes created by all revisions since then have been quantified as comparability ratios. Comparability ratios are derived by coding the mortality data based on the criteria of the new revision by the criteria of the old revision. A comparability ratio of 1.00 indicates that the same number of deaths was assigned to a particular cause or combination of causes, whether the earlier or the later revision was used. A ratio of 1.00 does not necessarily mean that no changes were made, however, as changes may have compensated for one another. A comparability ratio of less than 1.00 usually results from a decrease in the assignments of deaths to a cause in the later revision as compared to the earlier revision. A comparability ratio of more than 1.00 usually results from an increase in assignments of deaths to a cause in the later revision as compared to the earlier one (Klebba & Dolman, 1975). There are also separate comparability ratios for each 10-year age group (e.g., 15–24 years, 35–44 years); thus the total comparability ratio may be 1.00 for a specific cause of death, with the 15- to 24-year-olds having a ratio of 1.03, the 35- to 44-year-olds one of 0.97, and so on. The changes in the causes-of-death ratings for suicide and homicide

cide for the fourth revision and after are summarized in Table 4.1. As can be seen, the changes have been small.

Finally, mention should be made of a category introduced in 1968, in the eighth revision of the ICD: "[Deaths due to] Injuries undetermined whether accidentally or purposely inflicted" (i.e., category E980–E989). The initiation of this category may account to some extent for the fact that the comparability ratios for suicide, homicide, and accident data from the seventh to the eighth revision are all less than 1.00. For example, in 1975, 4,838 deaths were listed in E980–E989; in the same year, there were 27,063 suicides, 21,310 homicides, and 103,030 accidents.

Problems with Assessing the Population

The population statistics used for the derivation of U.S. national mortality rates are based on the census of the U.S. population conducted every 10 years, and on the interim estimates of the population (for the years when no census is taken), which are based on the preceding census. Three specific issues regarding population data are noteworthy.

TABLE 4.1. Changes in Cause-of-Death Ratings for Suicide and Homicide since the Fourth Revision of the *International Classification of Diseases*

Revisions	Suicide	Homicide
Fourth–fifth[a]	0%	−1.8%
Fifth–sixth[b]	1.00	1.00
Sixth–seventh[b]	1.03	1.00
Seventh–eighth[b]	0.9472	0.9969
Eighth–ninth[b]	1.0032	1.0057

Sources of data: Dunn and Shackley (1944), Faust and Dolman (1963, 1964, 1965), Klebba and Dolman (1975), National Center for Health Statistics (1980).

[a]Changes quantified as percentages.

[b]Changes quantified as comparability ratios.

First, beginning in 1933 the entire population in the United States was included in the mortality rates, whereas prior to 1933 only some states and cities were included. Second, during various wars there have been shifts of younger people overseas. Third, only estimates of the population are used during years in which no census is taken.

Prior to 1933, the population figures used by the federal government to derive national mortality statistics included only some of the states in the United States, as well as certain cities and metropolitan areas. This population aggregate, termed "death registration states," was increased by additional reporting states until 1933, when all the states were included (with Alaska added in 1959 and Hawaii in 1960). The composition and admission order of the death registration states can be found in *Death Rates by Age, Race, and Sex* . . . (1956). Thus, prior to 1933 the data represent only a sample of the U.S. patterns, whereas from 1933 on the entire population has been utilized. Therefore, in examining patterns of suicide and homicide in the United States, we emphasize the data for 1933 to the present rather than the more limited samples prior to 1933. In addition, from 1933 on any changes in mortality rates are statistically "significant," inasmuch as the data come from the entire population and not just samples.

The second population issue involves the location of the population used to derive rates. For U.S. data, our focus is on deaths occurring within the United States; it seemed advisable to limit the study to a specific country and location, and usually the U.S. population overseas is relatively small. The years of World War II and the Vietnam war accounted for the largest overseas shifts of youthful population during the time span of the present study.

The third problem involving the population figures concerns the decennial census method of determining the population. Because the census is only taken every 10 years, the population figures for determination of mortality rates are established not only for the year of the census but also for the 9 years following. The next census then represents something of a correction of the final years of the last decade (which were based on the census taken several years prior).

For example, the total U.S. population was calculated to be 214,649,000 for 1976, 216,332,000 for 1977, 218,228,000 for 1978, and 220,099,000 for 1979; that is, the increase in the population was estimated at slightly less than 2 million per year. The census of 1980 established the total U.S. population to be 227,236,000—an increase over the 1979 estimate of more than 7 million. The U.S. Bureau of the Census then had to go back and adjust the prior years, estimating a correction factor based on the new data.

A similar problem occurs with each census. The new census figures allow for more accurate estimates of the population for the prior 9 years. For example, the 1990 census figures allowed for revisions in the population estimate for 1981–1989. These revisions in turn lead to more accurate mortality rate derivation for the intervening years. For suicide and homicide, those changes in rates tend to be rather small, usually ranging from approximately 0.0 to 0.5 per 100,000 population. The current study utilizes the unpublished figures compiled by the National Center for Health Statistics for the years 1933–1959. For the years 1960–1979, the annual population figures published in *Vital Statistics of the United States* (National Center for Health Statistics, 1964–1983) have been utilized. For the years from 1980 to the most recent year for which data are available (usually 1990), unpublished data from the National Center for Health Statistics have been used.

In our definitions of race, the category "white" includes, in addition to those reported as white, persons reported to be Hispanic (including Mexican, Puerto Rican, and Cuban) (Klebba, 1979; National Center for Health Statistics, 1992). The categories "races other than white" or "all other" (referred to as "nonwhite" or "all other") consist of persons reported as African-American, Native American, Chinese, Japanese; other numerically small racial groups; and persons of mixed white and other races (Klebba, 1979). For example, the National Center for Health Statistics (1992) reported that in 1989, about 39,278,000 of the 248,239,000 people in the United States (or 15.8%) belonged to "races other than white." Of these 39,278,000 people, about 30,660,000 (or 78.1%) were African-American.

PATTERNS OF YOUTH SUICIDE
AND HOMICIDE

The methodologic concerns have been dealt with in detail above, but three issues should be reiterated here. First, underreporting is a problem with suicide data, and to a lesser extent with homicide data; many suicides and homicides are misclassified as accidents. Second, data classification comparability over time at the national level is good for both suicide and homicide. Third, national mortality data are used from 1933 to the most recent year for which data are available (usually 1990) in the United States. Data before 1933 are sample data only. Data from 1933 to the present are not sample data; they include all deaths by suicide and homicide recorded in the United States.

Suicide

To begin with, it is useful to explore the epidemiology of youth suicide in context by examining the numbers and rates of suicides for all age groups. Table 4.2 presents these suicide patterns by age, race, and sex for 1990 in the United States. With respect to actual numbers of deaths (see the top half of the table), 30,906 people died by suicide in 1990. With the exceptions of the 25–34 and 35–44 age groups, the highest *number* of suicides occurred among the 15–24 age group—4,869. The sharp increase over the number for the 5–14 age group (264) is particularly striking. Thus, in terms of numbers, the problem of suicide among adolescents and young adults commands serious attention. However, one reason why young people have so many suicides is that their population is currently so high in comparison to most other age groups. The bottom half of Table 4.2 demonstrates this by presenting the suicide rates for all age groups. The 15- to 24-year-olds have the lowest rate of any age group, with the exception of the far lower rate for the 5- to 14-year-olds. Suicide rates tend to increase with age, and the figures of 1990 represent a trend similar to those of previous years in

TABLE 4.2. Suicide Numbers and Rates by Age in Years, Race, and Sex, United States, 1990

	Total	0–1	1–4	5–14	15–24	25–34	35–44	45–54	55–64	65–74	75–84	85+
					Numbers							
Total	30,906	—	—	264	4,869	6,550	5,717	3,718	3,383	3,230	2,493	671
Male	24,724	—	—	195	4,160	5,339	4,424	2,836	2,563	2,546	2,099	554
Female	6,182	—	—	69	709	1,211	1,293	882	820	684	394	117
White male	22,448	—	—	165	3,569	4,625	4,008	2,630	2,428	2,435	2,046	534
White female	5,638	—	—	58	613	1,058	1,175	819	773	648	383	108
Nonwhite male	2,276	—	—	30	591	714	416	206	135	111	53	20
Nonwhite female	544	—	—	11	96	153	118	63	47	36	11	9
				Rates per 100,000 population								
Total	12.4	—	—	0.8	13.2	15.2	15.3	14.8	16.0	17.9	24.9	22.2
Male	20.4	—	—	1.1	22.0	24.8	23.9	23.2	25.7	32.2	56.1	65.9
Female	4.8	—	—	0.4	3.9	5.6	6.8	6.9	7.3	6.7	6.3	5.4
White male	22.0	—	—	1.1	23.2	25.6	25.3	24.8	27.5	34.2	60.2	70.3
White female	5.3	—	—	0.4	4.2	6.0	7.4	7.5	8.0	7.2	6.7	5.4
Nonwhite male	11.9	—	—	0.9	16.8	24.0	15.5	12.8	11.8	14.2	15.3	24.6
Nonwhite female	2.6	—	—	—	2.7	4.0	3.8	3.4	3.2	3.3	—	—

Note. Age not stated for 11 cases. A dash means no reported cases.

Source of data: National Center for Health Statistics, unpublished data, 1993.

43

the United States (Holinger, 1987). For all age groups, including adolescents, rates for whites are greater than those for nonwhites, and rates for males are higher than those for females. White males are at highest risk of suicide.

We now provide more detailed data on the trends in youth suicide. No deaths between birth and 4 years of age are recorded as suicides by the National Center for Health Statistics; recorded suicides for 5- to 9-year-olds are rare in the United States, usually about 0–10 per year during the 20th century. Suicide among 10- to 14-year-olds is also relatively rare, approximately 100–300 per year. A breakdown of the 1990 data for the 15–24 age group into 15–19 and 20–24 age groups is presented in Table 4.3. The older group has both greater numbers and higher rates of suicide. White males are at highest risk in both age groups.

Figures 4.1 and 4.2 present the longitudinal patterns of suicide rates for 15- to 19-year-olds, or middle to late adoles-

TABLE 4.3. Suicide Numbers and Rates by Race and Sex for 15–19 and 20–24 Age Groups, United States, 1990

	15- to 19-year-olds	20- to 24-year-olds
	Numbers	
Total	1,979	2,890
Male	1,656	2,504
Female	323	386
White male	1,422	2,147
White female	279	334
Nonwhite male	234	357
Nonwhite female	44	52
	Rates per 100,000 population	
Total	11.1	15.1
Male	18.1	25.7
Female	3.7	4.1
White male	19.3	26.8
White female	4.0	4.4
Nonwhite male	13.0	20.6
Nonwhite female	2.5	3.0

Source of data: See Table 4.2.

cents. The rates for 15- to 19-year-olds are much higher than for 10- to 14-year-olds, often five to ten times greater, with the number of suicides recently about 1,500–2,000. Period effects are apparent, with higher rates in the early 1930s (the Great Depression), lower rates during the 1940s (World War II), and increasing rates from the mid-1950s into the 1980s. Male rates are higher than female rates, and whites are higher than those for nonwhites. White males have the highest rates. As noted above, two recent controversial studies have suggested that misclassification errors account for some of the increase in suicide among 15- to 24-year-olds that occurred from the 1950s through the 1970s (Gist and Welch, 1989; Males, 1991).

Figures 4.3 and 4.4 present the longitudinal trends in suicide rates for 20- to 24-year-olds, or young adults. The rates for this group are approximately 1½ to 2 times those of the 15–19 group. Period effects are similar to the 15- to 19-year-olds, except that the rates of the 20- to 24-year-olds have tended to level off recently. The sex and race patterns for the two age groups are also similar: Males have higher rates than females, and whites higher rates than nonwhites.

The methods of suicide for the 15–19 and 20–24 age groups are similar (see Table 4.4). Firearms account for more than half the suicides for both age groups, with hanging being the second leading cause for both groups. With the exception of somewhat higher percentages of firearm suicides recently (Mościcki and Boyd, 1983–1985), no major shifts have occurred in these percentages since 1949, when methods of suicide began being reported in more detail (Holinger, 1978). Younger age groups (e.g., 10- to 14-year-olds) tend to have a somewhat lower proportion of suicide by firearms and a higher proportion by hanging.

Homicide

We can put the epidemiology of homicide among youth in context by examining the numbers and rates of homicides

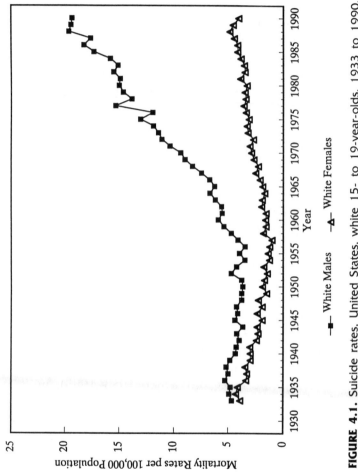
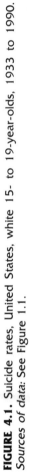

FIGURE 4.1. Suicide rates, United States, white 15- to 19-year-olds, 1933 to 1990. *Sources of data: See Figure 1.1.*

46

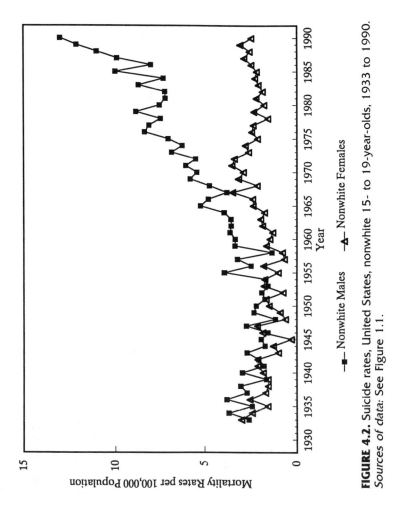

FIGURE 4.2. Suicide rates, United States, nonwhite 15- to 19-year-olds, 1933 to 1990. *Sources of data:* See Figure 1.1.

47

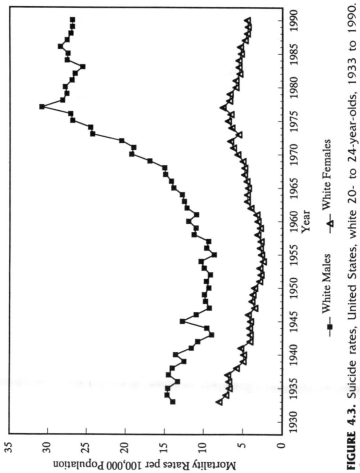

FIGURE 4.3. Suicide rates, United States, white 20- to 24-year-olds, 1933 to 1990. *Sources of data: See Figure 1.1.*

48

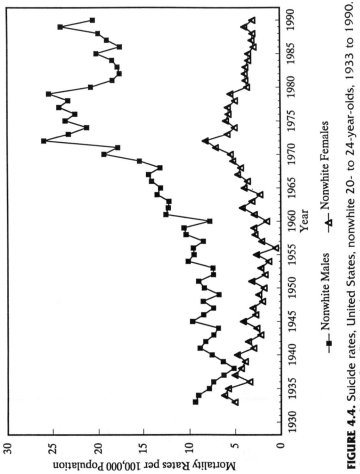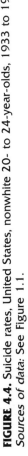

FIGURE 4.4. Suicide rates, United States, nonwhite 20- to 24-year-olds, 1933 to 1990. *Sources of data:* See Figure 1.1.

TABLE 4.4. Methods of Suicide for 15- to 24-Year-Olds, United States, 1990

	Total	Drugs (E950.0–E950.5)		Other solid or liquid substances (E950.6–E950.9)		Gases (E951–E952)		Hanging, strangulation, suffocation (E953)		Firearms (incl. handguns) (E955.0–E955.4)		Other means and late effects (E954; E955.5–E959)	
						15- to 19-year-olds							
Total	1,979	97	(4.9%)	5	(0.3%)	111	(5.6%)	365	(18.4%)	1,332	(67.3%)	69	(3.5%)
Male	1,656	43	(2.3%)	4	(0.2%)	89	(5.4%)	317	(19.1%)	1,151	(70.0%)	52	(3.1%)
Female	323	54	(16.7%)	1	(0.3%)	22	(6.8%)	48	(14.9%)	181	(56.0%)	17	(5.3%)
						20- to 24-year-olds							
Total	2,890	153	(5.3%)	13	(0.4%)	177	(6.1%)	546	(18.9%)	1,833	(63.4%)	168	(5.8%)
Male	2,504	70	(2.8%)	11	(0.4%)	154	(6.2%)	506	(20.2%)	1,627	(65.0%)	136	(5.4%)
Female	386	83	(21.5%)	2	(0.5%)	23	(6.0%)	40	(10.4%)	206	(53.4%)	32	(8.3%)

Source of data: National Center for Health Statistics, unpublished data, 1993. Percentage totals may not equal 100% because of rounding.

for all age groups (Table 4.5). The total number of homicides in the United States for 1990 was 24,932—or about
four-fifths the number of suicides. The number of homicides
among the 15–24 age group (7,354), however, was higher
than the number of suicides; in addition, the 15- to 24-year-
olds had the second greatest number of homicides, following
the 25- to 34-year-olds—similar to the pattern for suicide.
The bottom half of Table 4.5 gives the homicide rates for
1990. The rate for homicide among 15- to 24-year-olds
(19.9) is higher than that for suicide (13.2). The overall age
trends for homicide are quite different. Homicide rates tend
to peak in adolescence and early adulthood, unlike suicide
rates, which peak at greater ages. Thus, the 15- to 24-year-
olds have the highest homicide rates of any age group in the
United States. Male rates are higher than female rates, and—
as is not the case for suicide—nonwhite rates are far higher
than white rates. As with suicide, there is a marked increase
in homicide rates with the shift from the 5–14 to 15–24 age
group. Table 4.6 gives a further breakdown of the 1990
youth homicide numbers and rates. Again, as in the case of
suicide, the 20–24 age group has higher numbers and rates
of mortality. This breakdown also demonstrates that the
15–19 and 20–24 age groups have similar sex and race patterns, with males having higher rates than females, and nonwhites higher rates than whites.

Figures 4.5 and 4.6 demonstrate the longitudinal age,
race, and sex patterns for homicide rates among 15- to 19-
year-olds. As with suicide rates, the shift from the 10–14 to
15–19 age group produces a marked increase in homicide
rates: Rates for the older age group are approximately five to
ten times higher than for the younger group. Period effects
are readily discernible in the 15–19 group: higher rates in
the 1930s, lower rates in the 1940s and 1950s, increases from
the 1960s to the late 1970s and early 1980s, and a recent
leveling off (with the exception of the very recent increase
among 15- to 19-year-old nonwhite males). Male rates are
higher than female rates, and nonwhite rates are higher than
white rates. Nonwhite males have markedly higher rates than
the other race and sex groups.

TABLE 4.5. Homicide Numbers and Rates by Age in Years, Race, and Sex, United States, 1990

	Total	0–1	1–4	5–14	15–24	25–34	35–44	45–54	55–64	65–74	75–84	85+
					Numbers							
Total	24,932	332	378	512	7,354	7,643	4,417	1,892	1,055	682	430	139
Male	19,604	178	208	299	6,222	6,096	3,516	1,484	802	456	214	57
Female	5,328	154	170	213	1,132	1,547	901	408	253	226	216	82
White male	9,147	103	109	154	2,375	2,724	1,807	880	485	294	132	37
White female	3,006	78	81	113	590	769	512	289	179	163	158	51
Nonwhite male	10,457	75	99	145	3,847	3,372	1,709	604	317	162	82	20
Nonwhite female	2,322	76	89	100	542	778	389	119	74	63	58	31
					Rates per 100,000 population							
Total	10.0	8.4	2.6	1.5	19.9	17.7	11.8	7.6	5.0	3.8	4.3	4.6
Male	16.2	8.8	2.7	1.7	32.9	28.3	19.0	12.1	8.1	5.8	5.7	6.8
Female	4.2	8.0	2.4	1.2	6.3	7.2	4.8	3.2	2.3	2.2	3.4	3.8
White male	9.0	6.4	1.8	1.1	15.4	15.1	11.4	8.3	5.5	4.1	3.9	4.9
White female	2.8	5.1	1.4	0.8	4.0	4.3	3.2	2.6	1.8	1.8	2.8	2.5
Nonwhite male	54.8	18.1	6.6	4.1	109.1	96.5	63.5	37.6	27.8	20.8	23.6	24.6
Nonwhite female	11.1	18.8	6.1	2.9	15.5	20.3	12.6	6.3	5.1	5.8	10.0	17.3

Note. Age not stated for 98 cases.
Source of data: National Center for Health Statistics, unpublished data, 1993.

TABLE 4.6. Homicide Numbers and Rates by Race and Sex for 15–19 and 20–24 Age Groups, United States, 1990

	15- to 19-year-olds	20- to 24-year-olds
Numbers		
Total	3,042	4,312
Male	2,571	3,651
Female	471	661
White male	922	1,453
White female	248	342
Nonwhite male	1,649	2,198
Nonwhite female	223	310
Rates per 100,000 population		
Total	17.0	22.5
Male	28.0	37.5
Female	5.4	7.0
White male	12.5	18.1
White female	3.6	4.5
Nonwhite male	92.0	126.8
Nonwhite female	12.8	18.1

Source of data: See Table 4.5.

Figures 4.7 and 4.8 show the homicide rates for 20- to 24-year-olds. The rates again show an increase with age; they are approximately 1½–2 times higher for the 20–24 group than for the 15–19 group. Period effects are again clear, with higher rates in the 1930s; lower rates through the 1940s and 1950s, and into the 1960s; an increase in rates from the mid-1960s to the late 1970s and early 1980s; and a recent leveling off of rates. Male rates are higher than female rates, and nonwhite males are at far higher risk of homicide than the other groups.

The methods of homicide for 1990 are presented in Table 4.7. These methods are quite similar for the 15–19 and 20–24 age groups. Firearms account for about 75% of all homicides in both groups. For both groups, "All other [than handguns] and unspecified firearms" account for most deaths (approximately 70%–75%); "Cutting and piercing instruments" are next (approximately 10%–15%). There

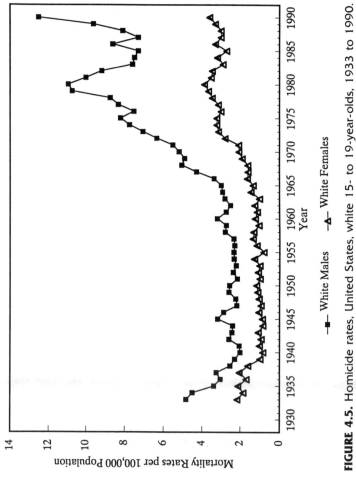

FIGURE 4.5. Homicide rates, United States, white 15- to 19-year-olds, 1933 to 1990. *Sources of data:* See Figure 1.1.

54

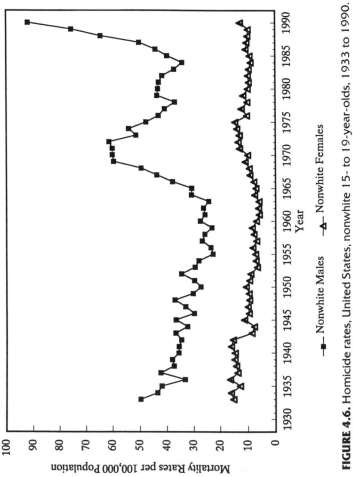

FIGURE 4.6. Homicide rates, United States, nonwhite 15- to 19-year-olds, 1933 to 1990. *Sources of data:* See Figure 1.1.

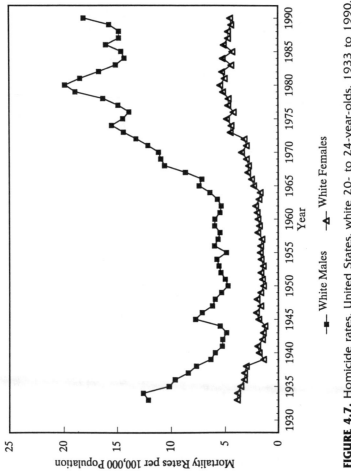

FIGURE 4.7. Homicide rates, United States, white 20- to 24-year-olds, 1933 to 1990. *Sources of data: See Figure 1.1.*

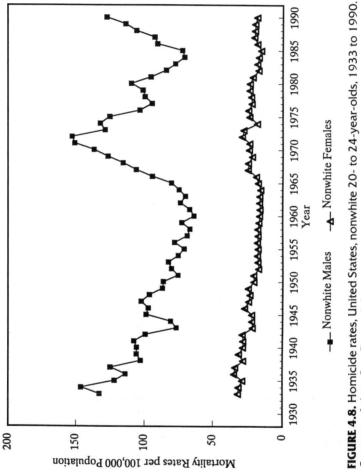

FIGURE 4.8. Homicide rates, United States, nonwhite 20- to 24-year-olds, 1933 to 1990. *Sources of data:* See Figure 1.1.

TABLE 4.7. Methods of Homicide for 15- to 24-Year-Olds, United States, 1990

		Handgun (E965.0)		All other and unspecified firearms (E965.1–E965.4)		Cutting and piercing instruments (E966)		Assault by all other means and late effects (E960–E964, E965.5–E965.9, E967–E969)		Legal execution (E978)	Other legal intervention (E970–E977)	
15- to 19-year-olds												
Total	3,042	181	(6.0%)	2,281	(75.0%)	321	(10.6%)	237	(8.0%)	0	22	(0.7%)
Male	2,571	155	(6.0%)	2,022	(78.6%)	247	(9.6%)	125	(4.9%)	0	22	(0.9%)
Female	471	26	(5.5%)	259	(55.0%)	74	(15.7%)	112	(23.8%)	0	0	
20- to 24-year-olds												
Total	4,321	224	(5.2%)	2,993	(69.4%)	651	(15.1%)	386	(9.0%)	0	58	(1.3%)
Male	3,651	194	(5.3%)	2,675	(73.3%)	516	(14.1%)	210	(5.8%)	0	56	(1.5%)
Female	661	30	(4.5%)	318	(48.1%)	135	(20.4%)	176	(26.6%)	0	2	(0.3%)

Source of data: National Center for Health Statistics, unpublished data, 1993. Percentage totals may not equal 100% because of rounding.

are differences between males and females, and these differences are consistent for both age groups. Females tend to have relatively fewer homicides by firearms, and relatively more by "Assault by all other means and late effects."

Suicide versus Homicide

It is also of interest to compare the longitudinal patterns of youthful suicide and homicide. Figures 4.9 and 4.10 show these trends from 1933 to 1990. It would appear that the period effects for suicide and homicide among youth are quite similar.

DISCUSSION

The epidemiologic variables for youth suicide and homicide—age, race, and sex—have been dramatically consistent over the 20th century in the United States. The rates for both suicide and homicide tend to increase throughout adolescence and early adulthood; youth suicide rates are higher for whites than for nonwhites, whereas nonwhites have higher homicide rates; and rates for males are higher than for females for both suicide and homicide. The reasons behind these descriptive data are still unclear and controversial. For example, the increase of rates with age may have multiple determinants. With increasing age in adolescence and young adulthood comes an increased frequency of various psychiatric disorders known to be related to suicide, such as schizophrenia, major depression, and bipolar disorder; increased age allows for increased cognitive and motor capacities to carry out suicide and homicide; increased separation from parents and family and added responsibilities for oneself (career, financial, etc.) occur with the transition from adolescence to young adulthood; and so on. Thus, with the increase of years during this period can come an increase in both internal vulnerabilities and external stresses for certain individuals. The reasons for the effects of race are even less

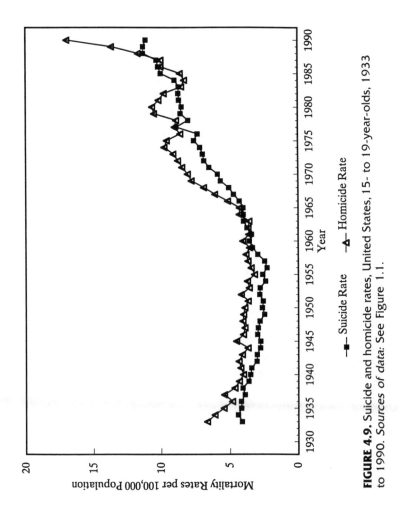

FIGURE 4.9. Suicide and homicide rates, United States, 15- to 19-year-olds, 1933 to 1990. Sources of data: See Figure 1.1.

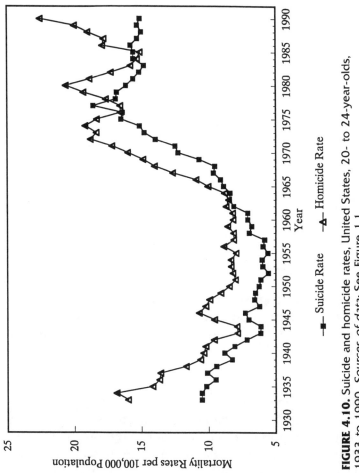

FIGURE 4.10. Suicide and homicide rates, United States, 20- to 24-year-olds, 1933 to 1990. *Sources of data:* See Figure 1.1.

— Suicide Rate   ▲ Homicide Rate

clear than those for age effects. The differences may be attributable more to poverty than to race per se; differences in child-rearing practices and genetics (degree of susceptibility to psychiatric disorders, such as bipolar illness) may also be involved. The difference in rates between males and females is also problematic: Socialization issues (e.g., greater career and financial pressures as perceived by males, and the increased action orientation of males) as well as biologic factors may help account for this.

The period effects for both youth suicide and homicide appear to be dominated by economic variables, times of declared war, and demographic shifts. With respect to the latter, the increasing number of 15- to 24-year-olds throughout the mid-1950s to the late 1970s seems to have contributed to the increase of rates during that time. The decrease in the proportion of 15- to 24-year-olds has been associated temporally with the leveling off of the rates; however, the increase in firearms and drugs over the past decade may be somewhat responsible for the rates' not decreasing since the peak of the 15–24 age cohort in the late 1970s.

Youth suicide and homicide have very similar age and sex patterns and very different race patterns. Strikingly, the numbers and trends over time are quite alike. This would suggest that, on an epidemiologic level, similar social pressures—such as the economy, war, and demographics—are responsible for fairly similar shifts in rates over time. This also suggests that interventions that effectively address these social pressures will have a positive impact on both youth suicide and homicide.

As described in Chapter 3, these epidemiologic data are of clinical importance. For example, suppose that a family physician sees an older white adolescent male who has a psychiatric history and guns at home; the young man came in to get help with his flu, but he also tells the doctor that he has been depressed. The physician, with a little epidemiologic knowledge and information, is immediately alerted to the potential suicidal risk and takes the necessary steps to start an appropriate evaluation. In turn, various clinical anecdotes and increasingly substantiated clinical findings can influence the direction of epidemiologic research. Such has been the case with recent studies documenting the character structure of suicidal adolescents, the importance of guns in the house, and the effect of drugs. Finally, epidemiologic data can dictate various public policy shifts that are crucial for lowering youth suicide and homicide rates (e.g., public education, gun control, etc.; see Chapters 7 and 8). These epidemiologic data include particularly the identification of risk (age, race, and sex) groups for which intervention efforts are most essential.

SUMMARY

Suicide rates for adolescents and young adults are lower than those for virtually any other age group, and youth homicide rates are higher than those for virtually any other ages, yet the long-term patterns of suicide and homicide among the young are similar. Suicide and homicide show an increase in rates with each 5-year age increment, from 10–14, to 15–19, to 20–24. The transition from 10–14 to 15–19 seems particularly important, with increases in rates occurring for suicide and homicide. In terms of race and sex, two patterns emerge: (1) Among the youthful age groups studied, males have higher rates than females for suicide and homicide; and (2) for all age groups, white rates are higher than nonwhite rates for suicide, whereas nonwhites have higher rates than whites for homicide.

Period effects tend to become clear from about 15 years and older, and these long-term trends are markedly similar for suicide and homicide. For suicide and homicide, rates tend to be high during the 1930s (economic depression) and lower during the 1940s (World War II); rates increase from the mid-1950s into the 1980s, with some leveling off for 20- to 24-year-olds.

CHAPTER FIVE

Demographic Patterns: United States

Demographic data suggest that population shifts among adolescents tend to be related to shifts in adolescent suicide and homicide rates (not simply numbers of deaths), with the potential prediction of these rates. A number of patterns emerge when we examine nonmortality data in this area. First, the bulk of evidence suggests that demographic shifts have some relationship to the increase in adolescent psychopathology, substance abuse, poor self-image, and crime in the United States during the 1960s and 1970s. Second, cross-cultural data also tend to support the influence of demographic variables in adolescent mortality and psychopathology. Third, evidence suggests that the nature of the demographic effect is either influenced by or mediated through economic variables. Fourth, adolescents may be especially susceptible to influences of particular events, such that a period effect may look like a cohort effect. Therefore, the major conceptual issue in determining the nature of the demographic influence may lie in the difficulty of distinguishing period effects from cohort effects. This is no small matter, as effective intervention and prevention strategies would depend upon such determinations.

Over the past decade, a number of clinical and epidemiologic advances have enhanced our understanding of youth suicide and homicide. In epidemiology, this enhancement has taken place primarily with respect to longitudinal trends. Specifically, new knowledge about such trends has resulted from studies on economic variables by Brenner (1971, 1973, 1979); research on demographic variables by Easterlin (1980); and examinations of cohort effects and demography by Klerman (1988, 1989), Hendin (1982), Murphy and Wetzel (1980), Solomon and Hellon (1980), Seiden and Freitas (1980), and ourselves (Holinger and Offer, 1981, 1982; Holinger et al., 1987).

Before we turn to these studies, however, a reminder regarding some definitions dealing with longitudinal trends is necessary. "Age effects" are changes in age-specific rates of mortality or illness over the life span of individuals (Holford, 1983). An age effect noted in Chapter 4 is that adolescents tend to have the lowest suicide rates of any age group other than children. "Period effects" are changes in rate of mortality or illness during a particular historical period (Holford, 1983). "Cohort effects" are differences in rates of mortality or illness among individuals defined by some shared temporal experience, such as year or decade or birth (Holford, 1983). Age, period, and cohort effects can interact with one another.

ECONOMIC VARIABLES: BRENNER'S RESEARCH

One of the major advances toward the understanding of longitudinal trends in suicide and homicide was made by Brenner (1971, 1973, 1979). Although many researchers have examined the relationships between suicide/homicide and the economy (e.g., see Durkheim, 1897/1951; Diekstra, 1990), Brenner was the first to demonstrate the importance of period effects in psychiatric epidemiology. He focused on a single variable—economic cycles—and related it to both mental hospitalizations and mortality. In his book *Mental Illness and the Economy* (1973), Brenner described the inverse relation between the state of the economy and mental illness that reaches a level of social visibility; he focused on unemployment rates and mental hospital admission rates over more than a century. Brenner concluded:

> First, it is clear that instabilities in the national economy have been the single most important source of fluctuation in mental-hospital admissions or admissions rates. Second, this

relationship is so consistent for certain segments of the society that virtually no major factor other than economic instability appears to influence variation in their mental hospitalization rates. Third, the relation has been basically stable for at least 127 years and there is considerable evidence that it has had greater impact in the last two decades. (1973, p. ix)

Brenner (1979) subsequently expanded his research in two important directions. First, he studied the relationship between economic patterns and morbidity and mortality, in addition to admissions to mental hospitals; second, he tested the model in England and Wales, in addition to the United States.

Data for the entire United States showed that indices of acute pathologic disturbances, including suicide and homicide, rose within a year of increased unemployment rates. Brenner next focused on chronic physical illnesses in which stress plays a role, especially cardiovascular disease. The earlier study of psychopathology suggested that increases in cardiovascular morbidity would follow increased unemployment within a few months, but that mortality would rise after a considerable time lag. The time lag was found to be 2–3 years for most age groups and both sexes.

Brenner then tested the model by analyzing the relations between trends in economic indices and mortality rates in England and Wales over the years 1936 through 1976. The following hypotheses were sustained for all age groups: Unemployment (indicating recession) was positively related to mortality rates, and long-term economic growth was inversely related to mortality rates. Suicide and homicide, for example, showed increases within a year of increasing unemployment, while cardiovascular mortality began to increase 2–3 years after increased unemployment, with the effect persisting for 10–15 years. The model appeared most appropriate for all cardiovascular disease and ischemic heart disease; it was largely effective for malignancy; and it was least appropriate for cerebrovascular disease.

Brenner concluded that the model had now been applied to England and Wales with results similar to analyses of

U.S. data for the same time span. He suggested that long-term economic growth also moderates the problems associated with economic instability: Management of the national economy improves, health care gets better in quality and availability, and more substantial income support can be provided for displaced workers and other participants in the labor force. Thus the long-term trend in economic growth (or prosperity) clearly acts to reduce mortality and certainly not to increase it, as had at times been suggested. Brenner also attempted to make the shift from his macroscopic data to a microscopic level; that is, he discussed the effect of an economic turndown on the individual. He noted that especially vulnerable in recessions are (1) those in industries whose goods or services are not essential; (2) the less skilled, who are the first to lose their jobs and the last to get their jobs back when the economy improves; and (3) those who find that over one turn in the business cycle their skills are no longer needed. For these groups (most often to be found in the lower socioeconomic classes), this lack of economic security is stressful: Social and family structures break down, and habits that are harmful to health are adopted. The effects manifest themselves both as acute psychopathological events (e.g., suicide) and as chronic diseases after a time lag of a few years.

Thus Brenner's work is of particular importance because of his emphasis on understanding longitudinal trends, as well as his findings that increased mortality is consistently related over time to economic downturns.

DEMOGRAPHIC VARIABLES: EASTERLIN'S RESEARCH

The second major recent contribution to our understanding of longitudinal trends in suicide and homicide is that of Easterlin (1980). Easterlin studied the "baby boomers" (i.e., those born after World War II). He investigated the impact of this cohort's size upon the cohort itself, as well as upon the rest of society in the United States. Although Easterlin's work did not directly address the topic of suicide and homicide, his work has profound implications for the present study for three reasons: (1) his emphasis on longitudinal trends; (2) his systematic introduction of the importance of demographic variables in understanding longitudinal trends in various social phenomena; and (3) his demonstration of the interaction of cohort and period effects (i.e., he showed that a large cohort may create economic problems [period effects]).

The Easterlin hypothesis maintains that there is a cause–effect relationship between birth cohort size and economic, social, educational, and political trends (Institute of Medicine, National Academy of Sciences, 1985b). Specifically, it correlates movements in birth rates and age-specific rates with particular behavioral phenomena. According to Easterlin, when the size of the birth cohort increases, it produces excessive competition for existing and limited resources and institutions, and results in "relative deprivation." Easterlin identified three broad social institutions through which the effects of cohort size operate: family, schools, and the labor market. Increases in the number of siblings and a shortening of the birth interval accompany increases in crude birth rate, and both are thought to result often in less parental attention and other negative effects because of crowding in the family. The incapacity of schools to absorb a larger cohort results in increased competition for the relatively limited supply of educational programs and extracurricular activities, as well as in larger classes and crowding. The relative deprivation felt by the students may reinforce their experiences in their families. Once members of the disadvantaged cohort reach the labor market, they are likely to encounter a large number of entrants competing for a relatively few opportunities (if the economy has not kept pace with demographic changes). Having come from similar situations in their families and schools, the individuals may not have the personal or educational resources needed to compete for the limited jobs. As a result, young adults from crowded cohorts tend to have higher unemployment rates, lower relative earnings, and less upward mobility than those from small cohorts.

Responses to the stresses and frustration of relative deprivation are variable, ranging from adaptive and corrective reactions to maladaptive and antisocial ones. In an effort to improve their economic conditions, members of a crowded cohort may exhibit adaptive behaviors, such as trying to improve their educational status, delaying marriage, reducing fertility, and having both spouses employed. On the other hand, these stresses may result in such antisocial behaviors as drug and alcohol abuse, crime, and suicide.

Several types of data that tend to support the Easterlin hypothesis, particularly drug abuse, suicide, and homicide rates. Between the mid-1950s and the late 1970s there was approximately a doubling in the size of the 15–24 age group. The proportion of this age group in the total population parallels the trend in drug use: Both peaked in the late 1970s. What has been observed is that from 1960–1979 there was a steady and dramatic increase in drug use, particularly marijuana, among young adults aged 18–24. Not only did the ratio of drug users to nonusers rise, but also the number of people reporting daily use increased significantly. Beginning in 1979, although the availability of substances increased, usage decreased. By 1984, rates of illicit drug use had decreased by half (Institute of Medicine, 1985b) and have continued to show a steady decline since then (Johnston et al., 1992). Similarly, suicide and homicide rates for 15- to 24-year-olds increased from the mid-1950s to the late 1970s. Subsequently, the rates of rise of suicide and homicide for that age group have leveled off, as has the proportion of 15- to 24-year-olds in the total U.S. population (Holinger et al., 1987). Data indicate that the rates of several other social problems, such as crime and divorce, seem to follow curves similar to those observed for substance abuse.

Easterlin (1980) noted that dramatic cohort effects emerged in the post-World War II period under a new environment of macroeconomic stabilization and immigration restriction, but he argued that the size of a cohort also affects the economy and is essentially the key independent variable. However, it would appear that there is not necessarily a clear time ordering of economic and demographic events; more likely, a complex set of interaction effects accounts for changing rates of sociomedical problems.

Distinguishing between a cohort effect and a period effect is difficult. Even trends that appear similar across several age groups may not clearly indicate a period effect, since it is possible for a cohort effect to operate specifically on its subjects and diffuse across other cohorts through intergenerational interaction. Likewise, trends that distinguish one age group from all others may not necessarily indicate a cohort effect. A period effect may have an impact on a particular cohort that will appear distinctive because of the circumstances or experiences of that cohort. For example, many adolescents may be especially susceptible to influences of particular events, such that a period effect may look like a cohort effect. The Vietnam war, for example, had an impact on the entire society but was perhaps most stressful for young adults. Thus period effects may have a greater impact on a particular age group than on others and act like cohort effects.

There are several competing schools of thought about how the size of a cohort affects behavior. Easterlin, as noted above, emphasized relative deprivation. A second possibility is a "social imitation" or "contagion" model, which attributes the impact of the size of the cohort to an interreactional mechanism; that is, the larger a young cohort is, the more opportunity there is for the development of a youth culture relatively insulated from the influence of older generations. The third cohort size theory, the "social control" theory, attributes the sociopathologic behaviors of the 1960s and 1970s to the inability of the conventional socialization mechanisms (school, police, family) to control a larger cohort. However, while the social control theory may provide an explanation for deviant behavior, it does not account for socially adaptive behavior (i.e., positive responses to stresses experienced by the cohort, such as deferring marriage and fertility). The three cohort size theories—the relative deprivation hypothesis, the contagion model, and the social control theory—posit different mechanisms through which size operates to influence rates of social problems.

The schema assumed by the Easterlin hypothesis suggests three possible points of intervention, each of which would require different approaches based on reasonable predictions. Intervention could occur prior to the arrival of an anticipated large cohort and would be of a preventive or controlling nature. For example, if a large cohort is anticipated, and it is considered desirable to control the increase in cohort size, this might be approached by offering financial incentives to either defer or deter marriage and/or fertility. Second, if an increased cohort size leads to increased competition for established limited resources, policy response could be to increase or alter the available resources, such that the opportunity structure is more suited to meet an increased demand. This could occur at an early period in the reinforcing cycle (e.g., at the adolescent stage by enlarging schools or increasing the student–teacher ratio) or at a later point in the cycle, when the subject cohort is entering the labor market. The third type of intervention would involve the building of appropriate social support systems (counseling centers, etc.) to respond to the increased stress resulting from relative deprivation, and could be implemented at any stage in the cycle (e.g., increasing support systems before stress-related behavior disorders occur or helping people cope with their problems after they are manifested) (Institute of Medicine, 1985b). To date, most interventions have been after-the-fact attempts to deal with obvious problems.

DEMOGRAPHY AND NONMORTALITY MEASURES

In addition to Easterlin's work, two other studies deserve mention because of their attempts to clarify the influence of population shifts on nonmortality measures. Offer et al. (1988) explored the relationship between demographic and nonmortality variables from a longitudinal perspective, using the Offer Self-Image Questionnaire (OSIQ). These researchers found that 1970s adolescents fared the worst, that 1960s adolescents fared the best, and that 1980s adolescents fared the next best. The adolescents of the 1960s were the least depressed, least fearful about their future, and least impulsive; they also had the best social and interpersonal relationships and the highest ethical values. The adolescents in the 1970s were worse off in each of these ways. Interestingly, the authors noted that not one of the 130 OSIQ items contradicted the idea that the adolescents from the 1960s were better off than those in the 1970s or 1980s. Offer at al. (1988) suggested that these results could best be accounted for by the demographic shifts described above and their socioeconomic consequences.

Another investigator who has studied adolescents and demographic and nonmortality variables is Klerman (1988, 1989). Klerman summarized large-sample family studies, community epidemiologic surveys, and other data for both the United States and other countries. Klerman stated that the evidence seems to suggest that the "baby boomers" had as adolescents (and continue to have) increased rates of depression and other related illnesses, including drug abuse and alcoholism. Klerman (1988, 1989) described seven trends documented in the literature: (1) an increase in the prevalence of depression, particularly since World War II; (2) a marked increase in depression among those in cohorts born after World War II, adults now in their 30s and 40s; (3) an earlier age of onset of depression through the 20th century; (4) relative to previous older cohorts, an apparent decrease in depression among adults in cohorts born before 1920, individuals now in their 60s and 70s; (5) an effect for family aggregation resulting in increased risk of depression in the first-degree relatives of ill patients, suggestive of, but not conclusively establishing, genetic transmission for certain forms of depression; (6) an increase in risk for females in rates of depression across all cohorts; (7) evidence of a period effect interacting with gender and age, such that young females were at greatest risk during the 1960s and 1970s. Klerman noted the possibility of environmental risk factors' being involved (e.g., changes in nutrition, possible role of viruses, or effects of unknown depressogenic chemical agents in water or air), but appeared to favor a cohort or period effect as accounting for the increases in depression and other psychopathology among "baby boomer" youth.

COHORT ANALYSES

Another type of research that has recently been employed to examine demographic effects is the "cohort analysis." A cohort analysis identifies a cohort born during a certain time frame (e.g., 1950–1954) and follows this cohort over time with respect to morbidity, mortality, and so on. Although cohort analyses involve demographic variables, they are somewhat different from Easterlin's work, which followed a cohort ("baby boomers") specifically because of its relatively large size.

Cohort analyses have recently been used specifically to provide data to demonstrate the increase of suicide rates among the young (Solomon and Hellon, 1980; Murphy and Wetzel, 1980). Solomon and Hellon (1980) studying Alberta, Canada, during the years 1951–1977, identified 5-year age cohorts and followed the suicide rates as the cohorts aged. Suicide rates increased directly with age, regardless of gender. Once a cohort entered the 15–19 age range with a high rate of suicide, the rate for the cohort remained consistently high as it aged. Murphy and Wetzel (1980) found the same phenomenon (in reduced magnitude) in birth cohorts of much greater size in the United States. Not only did each successive birth cohort start with a higher suicide rate, but at each successive 5-year interval it had a higher rate than the preceding cohort had at that age. Goldney and Katsikitis (1983) reported similar findings in a cohort analysis of suicide rates in Australia. However, they noted some differences between their findings and those of the American and Canadian studies, based on the introduction in Australia of legislation that restricted the prescription of sedatives. Thus, they suggested that although there might be early and long-lasting cohort effects on successive birth cohorts, the suicide rates could also be influenced by changing environmental factors more immediately related to the suicide itself.

Klerman (1988, 1989) reported findings similar to those of the studies described above in his research on depressed patients: The cohort analyses indicated an increase in depression among the young for successive birth cohorts.

Other types of studies have given mixed support to the general idea that changes in population may be related to suicide rates. For example, Wechsler (1961) found that rapidly growing communities tended to produce significantly higher rates of suicide. Gordon and Gordon's (1960) earlier results tended to be consistent with Wechsler's data. Klebba (1975) discussed the increase of homicide among the young and suggested, but did not systematically pursue, an etiologic connection between the rising rates of homicide and increases in the adolescent population over the past two decades. On the other hand, Levy and Herzog (1974, 1978) and Herzog et al. (1977) found negative or insignificant correlations between population density and crowding on the one hand, and suicide rates on the other.

Finally, a different type of study has also tended to support a relationship between population changes and suicide rates. We (Holinger and Offer, 1981, 1982; Holinger et al., 1987) and Hendin (1982) studied the 15–24 age group from the early 1900s to the present. Both Hendin and we noted that increases and decreases in the proportion of 15- to 24-year-olds were accompanied by increases and decreases, respectively, in their suicide and homicide rates. These studies differed from the cohort studies in that they followed a specific age group over time (i.e., 15- to 24-year-olds), as opposed to following a particular birth cohort as it aged. This research is described in more detail in the next section of this chapter.

There are similarities and differences between the "population model" studies (Hendin, 1982; Holinger and Offer, 1981, 1982; Holinger et al., 1987) and the cohort effect studies. The similarities are found in the emphasis on recent increases in suicide rates among the younger age groups. The differences are found in the predictive aspects. The cohort studies suggested that the suicide rates for the age groups under study would continue to increase as they were followed over time. Implicitly, the cohort studies convey that the suicide rates for the younger age groups will continue to increase as each new 5-year adolescent cohort comes into being. The predictions generated by the population model are different. The population model suggests that the suicide and homicide rates for the younger age groups will begin leveling off and decreasing, inasmuch as the population of younger people has started to decrease. As discussed below, the current decreased rate of rise or leveling off of suicide and homicide rates among 15- to 24-years olds since the late 1970s tends to support the population model. Murphy et al. (1986), in their study of suicide in England and Wales, also presented data that cast doubt on the usefulness of cohort analyses in predicting the future rates of cohorts from their early behavior.

THE POPULATION MODEL

Findings Based on the Model

The "population model" is a term used to describe relationships between mortality rates for a specific age group (e.g., 15- to 24-year-olds) and the population shifts within that same age group over time. That is, the age group stays the same, but the subjects change over time. Research using the population model is different from cohort studies, which pick a group of people with date of birth or some historical event in common, and then follow this same group of subjects as they age. The distinction between the population model research and cohort studies is straightforward: Although cohort studies do not necessarily examine the relationship between mortality rates and population shifts, they may explore this variable, as in the case of Easterlin's (1980) work with the "baby boom" cohort.

The findings of the population model research have been presented in a series of papers (Holinger and Offer, 1981, 1982, 1984; Holinger et al., 1987, 1988) and are described briefly here. The population model relates the large shifts in the adolescent population to the suicide and homicide rates among youth. The findings have shown that as the proportion of adolescents increases, the suicide and homicide rates in that age group also increase. It should be stressed that this increase is not a simple increase in the numbers of suicides and homicides (which would obviously be expected to increase with an increase in population); it is an increase in the *rates* (deaths per 100,000 population). Decreases in the adolescent population have been related to decreases in the suicide and homicide rates of youth. The opposite trend has been found for adult age groups. That is, as the proportion of adults increases (or decreases), their suicide and homicide rates have decreased (or increased, respectively). These results are statistically significant for time-series analyses of various age groups over 50 years of longitudinal data in the United States. For example, Figures 5.1 and 5.2 present these patterns for 15- to 24-year-olds and 35- to 44-year-olds, respectively. As can be seen, with the exception of the past few years, there is a positive relationship between shifts in the youthful population and their suicide and homicide rates, and an inverse relationship between the population shifts for adults and their suicide and homicide rates (Holinger et al., 1987).

The national patterns have also been studied over time on a regional basis (i.e., for individual states in the United States). Those states with a high proportion of youth showed high rates of youth suicide and homicide, whereas those with a low proportion had low rates. Contrariwise, states with a high proportion of adults had low rates of suicide and homicide among adults, where those with a low proportion of adults had high adult rates of suicide and homicide (Holinger and Lester, 1991).

The explanations for these findings have included issues of competition and failure, and are consistent both with Easterlin's (1980) relative deprivation hypothesis and with Barker and Gump's studies of large and small schools (Barker and Gump, 1964; Barker, 1968). As the number of adolescents increases, there are more competitors for the same number of positions: jobs, positions on varsity sports

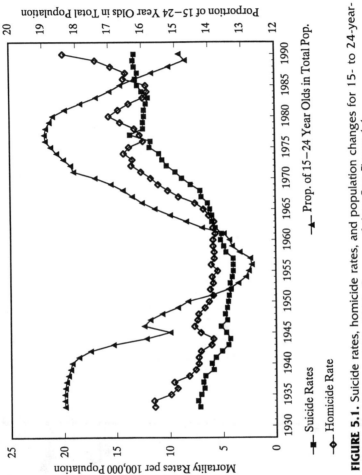

FIGURE 5.1. Suicide rates, homicide rates, and population changes for 15- to 24-year-olds, United States, 1933–1990. *Sources of data:* See Figure 1.1.

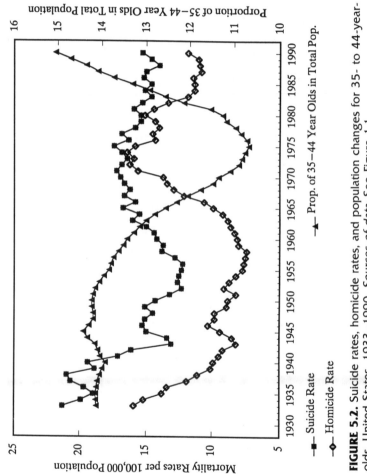

FIGURE 5.2. Suicide rates, homicide rates, and population changes for 35- to 44-year-olds, United States, 1933–1990. *Sources of data:* See Figure 1.1.

78

teams, places in the freshman classes of good colleges, access to various social and medical services (e.g., school counselors to help adolescents with problems, probation officers, vocational counselors, psychiatric services), and so on. The increased adolescent population and increased competition for such places result in an increased number of adolescents who fail to get these positions. Thus, with an increased adolescent population (some of whom will be psychologically and/or biologically vulnerable), relatively more adolescents will fail to achieve their goals, will see themselves as failures, will become depressed, will engage in riskier behaviors, will be unable to re-establish a balance in their self-esteem equilibrium, and will begin a downhill slide resulting eventually in suicide or homicide.

How might we understand this process psychologically? Inasmuch as external social pressures do not affect all youth equally, the concept of youthful individuals' being "at risk" or "internally vulnerable" is important. Particularly important for infants and children are the needs and capacities for self-soothing, tension regulation, and self-esteem regulation, which under ideal circumstances become increasingly internalized and less dependent on, and subject to, the external world. Of course, many patients—perhaps particularly those who become suicidal—do not internalize these functions, and this leads to a variety of clinical phenomena. For instance, one often sees in suicidal patients decreased capacities for tension regulation and self-soothing. Rapid regressions and fragmentation occur in the face of frustrations, slights, and failures, as patients suffer disruptions in their narcissistic homeostasis. When an unusually large cohort exists, as happened among adolescents from the late 1950s to the late 1970s, the entire system appears stressed and overburdened on a number of different levels. For instance, parents have too many children, schools have too many pupils, businesses have too many job applicants, and the mental health care system has too many patients. In these instances, the psychologically vulnerable children are increasingly at risk as the environment is less and less able to provide the external sources of self-esteem, treatment opportunities, and other needs that might aid in preventing a suicidal or homicidal outcome. Sophisticated studies of the beneficial effects of small schools versus large schools by Barker and Gump (1964) and Barker (1968) have demonstrated how this may occur operationally.

In addition, the members of the 15–24 age group may be the least powerful and attractive force in society with respect to political pressure, jobs, and so on. By contrast, the adults in the 35–64 age groups are much more powerful politically and are much more attractive employees because of more experience and schooling. Thus, the population increases in the adult groups may lead not so much to increased competition and failure, but rather to more economic benefits (greater and more successful pressure on government and union leaders to enlarge the job market, obtain more health services, etc.). Therefore, suicide and homicide rates should decrease with the increased population ratio in adults.

These data can also be related specifically to Brenner's (1971, 1979) and Easterlin's (1980) work. Brenner demonstrated that indicators of economic instability and insecurity such as unemployment were associated over time with higher mortality rates, including suicide and homicide. His explanation for this association was that lack of economic security is stressful; social and family structures break down, and habits that are harmful to health are adopted. The data showed that suicide and homicide are parallel over time, and Brenner's model suggests a reason for the parallel rates: economic cycles. Easterlin (1980) has related population increases in specific age groups to worsening economic conditions in those age groups. Turner et al. (1981) tended to support Brenner's (1980) work, reporting increases (and decreases) in economic well-being among adolescents and young adults that correspond clearly to the decreases (and increases, respectively) in the youthful population data presented in the population model.

Easterlin's and Brenner's work makes it possible to integrate demographic and economic variables with time trends for suicide and homicide. Although the relationship between the economy and mortality rates is well documented (i.e., bad economic conditions are related to higher mortality rates), we cannot predict future mortality rates from this relationship, inasmuch as without considering population variables we do not know what economic conditions will be like in the future. On the other hand, the population model suggested here may allow future predictions not only of suicide and homicide rates but also of economic conditions for certain age groups, because the population shifts for specific age groups are known years ahead. Finally, this predictive cycle becomes even more complete when we consider that the birth rate in the United States (which is responsible for most of the relevant population changes) tends to be inversely related to economic changes in the United States (i.e., high and low birth rates correspond to good and bad economic conditions, respectively). Thus, the interrelationship of these variables becomes clear: From the birth rate come relevant population changes; these population changes appear to influence economic conditions (i.e., unemployment); economic conditions and the population changes tend to influence not only changes in suicide and homicide rates but also changes in the birth rates, thus completing the cycle. Breaking into the cycle and extracting data on population changes create the potential for prediction of suicide and homicide rates.

Predictions Generated by the Model

One of the tasks of science is setting up hypotheses that can be falsified. The data have shown that increases (and decreases) in the proportion of adolescents in the United States are accompanied by increases (and decreases, respectively) in youth suicide and homicide rates. The potential for prediction of time trends of adolescent rates exists with these findings, inasmuch as the proportion of adolescents in the population can be determined years in advance. On the basis of this model, we have predicted that after the high rates in the late 1970s, the youth suicide and homicide rates will level off and decrease throughout the 1980s and into the mid-1990s, at which time another increase will begin (Holinger et al., 1988). Some of these predicted trends have been sustained: Suicide rates among 20- to 24-year-olds (see Figure 5.3) have tended to level off, and the rise of homicide rates from the mid-1970s to 1990 is far less than the rise from 1960 to the mid-1970s. Contrary to the predictions, the suicide and homicide rates among 15- to 19-year-olds (see Figure 5.4) have increased since 1985 or so, but there was a statistically significant decrease in the rate of rise from the 1970s to the mid-1980s (Holinger et al., 1988). Needless to say, several decades of data will be necessary for researchers to assess the actual value of this model and determine whether or not the hypothesis is falsified. Although we have focused on a single variable (population shifts) because of its predictive possibilities, variables such as period effects (e.g., economic conditions), divorce rates, drug use, firearm availability, and others should also be noted.

The predictions generated by the population model have also been compared with the predictions of the cohort studies (Holinger and Offer, 1989). As noted above, the cohort studies seem to suggest that the suicide and homicide rates for younger age groups will continue to increase as each new 5-year adolescent cohort comes into being. The population model's predictions are different: Suicide and homicide rates for younger age groups will begin leveling off and decreasing, because the population of younger people has started to decrease. In addition, the population model suggests that as the current group of youngsters gets older, suicide rates will increase less than predicted by the cohort studies. It is well known that male suicide rates increase with age in the United States, whereas female rates increase with age until about 65 years old and then decrease (Kramer et al., 1972). Therefore one would expect an increase in suicide rates with age, consistent with this long-established pattern. However, the current groups of adolescents and young adults make up an unusually large proportion of the U.S. population. The population model states that the larger the proportion of the adults in the population, the lower their suicide rates will be. Thus, the population model predicts

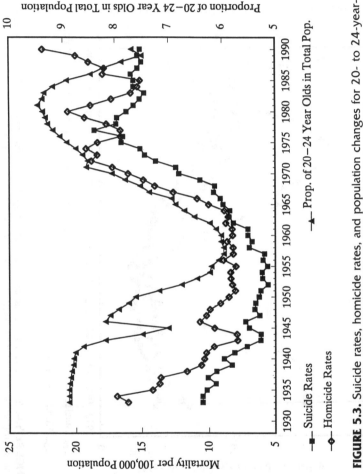
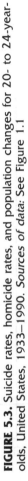

FIGURE 5.3. Suicide rates, homicide rates, and population changes for 20- to 24-year-olds, United States, 1933–1990. *Sources of data:* See Figure 1.1

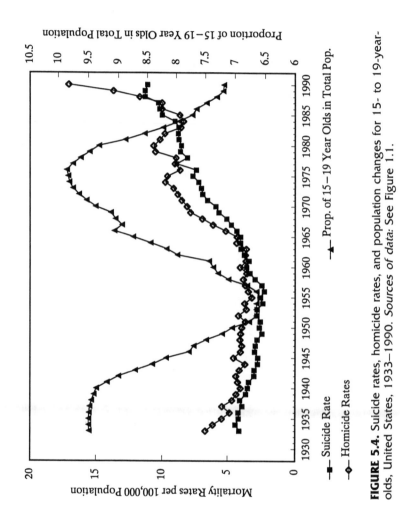

FIGURE 5.4. Suicide rates, homicide rates, and population changes for 15- to 19-year-olds, United States, 1933–1990. *Sources of data:* See Figure 1.1.

that suicide rates for the adult populations will decrease over the next several decades, compared with adult rates in the past; this is consistent with the movement of the "baby boom" population increase through those adult age groups. This is not to say that the rates for the older groups will be lower than for the younger groups, but rather that the older groups of the future may be expected to have lower suicide rates than the older groups of the past.

CHAPTER SIX

A Cross-Cultural Perspective

Cross-cultural data indicate that suicide rates for adolescents in the United States fall approximately in the upper third of the several countries studied, whereas homicide rates among adolescents in the United States are higher than in virtually all other countries. In addition, the relationship between demographic variables and adolescent suicide and homicide rates in the United States is found in some, but not all, countries studied.

The data on suicide and homicide in the United States raise some important questions. For example, how do U.S. rates compare to rates of other countries? Are the age patterns found in the United States similar to those of other countries? Are population shifts related to youthful suicide and homicide rates in other countries, as they may be in the United States? The purpose of this chapter is twofold. First, we describe the mortality rates for suicide and homicide in 20 countries representing several cultures, and compare these patterns with those from the United States. In this way, we may be able to assess which features of the patterns appear to be culture-bound and which may be universal. Second, we explore the relationship between demographic variables and various mortality and nonmortality measures among selected countries other than the United States.

SUICIDE AND HOMICIDE IN 20 COUNTRIES

This section presents cross-cultural data on suicide and homicide in 20 countries: Austria, Bulgaria, Canada,

Czechoslovakia, Denmark, England/Wales, Finland, France, Greece, Hungary, Japan, Mexico, Norway, Poland, Portugal, Switzerland, the United States, Uruguay, the former West Germany, and Yugoslavia. The data presented are national mortality data for 1990; these data have also been compared to those for other years, and this analysis has yielded patterns similar to those for the 1990 data, with only slight variation in the rankings of various countries. The major methodologic problems in cross-cultural comparisons of suicide and homicide rates among the young are classification changes over time and misclassification of cases, especially underreporting, for each country (Brooke, 1974; Klebba, 1975).

Tables 6.1 and 6.2 give 1990 suicide and homicide rates, respectively, for the 20 countries in rank order, broken down by age and sex. In order to put the cross-cultural rates for youth in perspective, we first examine the trends for all ages. For suicide, Hungary, Finland, and Austria have the highest rates; England/Wales, Greece, and Mexico have the lowest. Suicide rates for the United States fall approximately in the bottom third of those for the 20 countries. For homicide, Mexico and the United States have by far the highest rates; Denmark, Japan, and England/Wales have the lowest. Sex patterns are similar for suicide and homicide, with virtually all countries and age groups showing higher rates for males (the exception being homicide among younger females in some countries). Age patterns, however, show differences between suicide and homicide. For instance, for suicide the age trends are similar to those of the United States: The rates increase with age (with some countries showing a slight decrease of rates for older women). That is, the lowest rates are found in the youngest age groups. For homicide, the pattern is more complicated, with many countries showing patterns similar to those of the United States (i.e., the higher homicide rates are found in the 15–24, 25–34, and 35–44 age groups).

In examining the suicide and homicide rates for 15- to 24-year-olds in the 20 countries, we can see a number of patterns. First, for youth suicide, Finland, Switzerland, and Austria have the highest rates; Mexico and Greece have the lowest. The suicide rates for U.S youth are in the upper third

TABLE 6.1. Suicide Rates by Age and Sex for 20 Countries, 1990

Country		All ages	0–1	1–4	5–14	15–24	25–34	35–44	45–54	55–64	65–74	75+
Hungary	M	59.9	—	—	2.5	20.1	56.0	79.5	99.6	90.2	97.3	196.6
	F	21.4	—	—	0.8	8.2	11.8	20.3	29.9	28.8	37.1	75.6
Finland	M	49.3	—	—	1.2	50.9	64.1	68.1	63.7	56.3	49.6	90.1
	F	12.4	—	—	—	11.0	12.9	17.7	17.4	19.8	16.6	10.2
Austria	M	34.8	—	—	0.2	25.0	32.7	37.3	47.7	44.0	66.8	107.6
	F	13.4	—	—	0.5	5.5	8.4	13.9	16.5	20.8	22.0	35.5
Denmark	M	32.2	—	—	1.0	14.1	26.7	44.5	53.0	43.7	47.3	76.7
	F	16.3	—	—	—	4.0	6.9	18.4	27.3	31.5	30.0	32.2
Switzerland	M	31.5	—	—	—	24.8	33.2	32.2	39.0	42.7	51.6	86.8
	F	12.7	—	—	1.1	6.3	10.9	12.8	19.6	16.3	23.1	23.5
France	M	29.6	—	—	0.4	14.1	30.6	37.2	41.1	38.3	47.1	105.9
	F	11.1	—	—	0.1	4.4	9.1	11.8	16.4	18.1	18.5	25.6
Czechoslovakia	M	27.3	—	—	0.6	12.2	25.4	36.0	48.9	41.1	54.3	98.6
	F	8.9	—	—	0.2	4.3	6.4	8.8	11.3	13.8	19.7	29.4
Norway	M	23.3	—	—	1.5	22.1	28.0	29.7	28.3	34.1	34.3	30.9
	F	8.0	—	—	—	6.3	6.1	10.3	14.1	12.8	13.9	7.9
West Germany	M	22.4	—	—	0.4	15.0	21.3	22.2	28.2	31.0	34.6	72.2
	F	9.6	—	—	0.1	4.5	6.9	7.6	11.4	12.8	17.1	23.7
Poland	M	22.0	—	—	1.0	16.2	30.4	33.0	38.4	36.3	28.0	27.3
	F	4.5	—	—	0.2	2.8	4.3	6.0	7.4	8.7	7.2	7.4

Yugoslavia	M	21.6	—	—	1.1	9.6	17.2	23.2	34.1	40.3	56.5	97.3
	F	9.2	—	—	0.5	3.6	5.1	8.6	13.3	16.9	23.7	32.3
Bulgaria	M	20.7	—	—	2.2	13.9	17.2	17.6	24.2	27.6	43.5	97.1
	F	8.8	—	—	0.3	4.2	4.9	6.4	8.1	11.7	23.1	38.9
Japan	M	20.4	—	—	0.4	9.2	18.4	21.5	32.0	32.5	36.6	62.9
	F	12.4	—	—	0.2	4.7	9.0	9.2	15.0	17.6	25.3	48.6
Canada	M	20.4	—	—	1.2	24.6	29.6	26.7	23.4	22.6	20.7	32.4
	F	5.2	—	—	0.4	5.0	6.4	9.0	7.4	5.4	5.9	4.2
United States	M	20.4	—	—	1.1	22.0	24.8	23.9	23.2	25.7	32.2	57.9
	F	4.8	—	—	0.4	3.9	5.6	6.8	6.9	7.3	6.7	6.0
Uruguay	M	16.6	—	—	1.1	13.4	12.5	19.8	24.8	30.2	29.9	71.2
	F	4.2	—	—	1.1	2.9	3.6	3.7	4.1	3.0	16.8	10.0
Portugal	M	13.5	—	—	0.7	7.4	14.0	11.9	15.9	22.0	30.2	57.8
	F	4.5	—	—	—	3.1	3.6	3.5	5.8	5.7	8.3	15.9
England/Wales	M	12.1	—	—	0.1	11.7	16.0	17.1	16.4	13.3	13.6	19.4
	F	3.7	—	—	—	2.0	3.8	4.5	5.1	5.3	6.1	6.2
Greece	M	5.5	—	—	0.4	5.2	6.3	5.5	5.3	7.1	7.1	17.4
	F	1.5	—	—	—	1.1	1.5	0.9	3.0	2.1	2.6	2.4
Mexico	M	3.9	—	—	0.4	5.0	6.1	6.7	6.0	7.4	10.0	17.8
	F	0.7	—	—	0.1	1.2	0.9	0.8	0.8	1.2	0.9	0.8

Note. A dash means no reported cases.

Sources of data: For all countries except United States: World Health Organization, *World Health Statistics Annual 1992.* Geneva, Switzerland: World Health Organization, 1993. For United States: National Center for Health Statistics, unpublished data, 1993.

TABLE 6.2. Homicide Rates by Age and Sex for 20 Countries, 1990

Country		All ages	0–1	1–4	5–14	15–24	25–34	35–44	45–54	55–64	65–74	75+
Mexico	M	30.7	5.8	2.2	3.0	35.5	55.5	55.0	56.0	48.4	46.5	54.0
	F	3.6	4.8	1.8	1.4	3.6	4.4	4.9	4.2	5.4	6.5	14.9
United States	M	16.2	8.8	2.7	1.7	32.9	28.3	19.0	12.1	8.1	5.8	5.9
	F	4.2	8.0	2.4	1.2	6.3	7.2	4.8	3.2	2.3	2.2	3.5
Uruguay	M	7.0	—	0.9	0.4	5.7	8.8	12.6	10.2	9.4	9.3	9.6
	F	2.0	3.6	1.0	0.4	3.3	2.7	1.6	0.6	3.0	0.8	4.4
Bulgaria	M	5.1	5.6	—	0.5	5.6	8.8	7.2	7.2	4.3	3.0	5.6
	F	1.5	2.0	—	1.0	0.6	2.8	1.7	1.7	0.7	1.7	3.6
Finland	M	5.0	5.9	0.8	0.3	3.6	5.1	8.1	9.1	5.0	4.6	3.5
	F	1.6	3.1	—	—	2.8	2.1	2.2	1.7	1.9	1.3	—
Hungary	M	4.2	6.2	1.6	0.7	1.6	4.8	6.7	6.9	4.9	4.5	8.7
	F	2.1	4.9	1.7	0.6	1.1	2.8	2.9	2.9	1.5	1.6	3.8
Poland	M	4.1	6.1	0.2	0.4	2.3	5.2	7.4	6.7	5.0	5.8	6.0
	F	1.8	5.3	0.3	0.5	0.5	1.8	2.2	2.8	2.7	2.5	5.2
Yugoslavia	M	2.9	2.3	0.6	0.2	2.2	4.6	4.7	3.3	3.6	3.6	2.9
	F	1.1	1.9	0.1	0.2	0.6	1.0	2.0	1.1	1.4	1.7	1.6
Canada	M	2.7	2.4	1.3	0.5	3.5	4.4	3.2	3.0	2.1	2.3	1.3
	F	1.5	1.0	1.2	0.6	1.7	2.6	1.7	1.3	0.7	1.4	0.8
Portugal	M	2.5	6.7	0.4	—	2.4	3.2	3.8	2.4	4.2	2.7	2.6
	F	0.9	7.1	—	0.4	0.4	1.2	1.1	1.8	1.2	0.2	0.9

Czechoslovakia	M	2.3	5.6	0.2	0.2	1.3	3.2	3.8	2.0	3.2	3.1	6.1
	F	1.6	7.8	0.5	0.5	1.5	1.8	2.3	0.9	1.7	1.6	3.4
Austria	M	1.9	12.9	1.1	0.4	1.8	2.2	2.4	2.7	1.3	—	2.3
	F	1.4	4.5	1.2	1.4	0.9	1.6	1.4	0.8	1.9	1.5	1.6
Norway	M	1.8	—	0.9	0.4	2.1	2.1	1.9	3.1	2.1	1.7	0.9
	F	0.6	—	0.9	—	0.6	1.3	1.0	0.9	—	—	—
Switzerland	M	1.6	2.3	2.5	0.5	1.5	2.4	1.8	1.8	0.9	2.2	0.6
	F	1.3	2.4	2.0	0.8	1.1	1.1	2.0	2.1	1.7	0.3	0.7
Greece	M	1.5	—	—	0.1	1.6	3.1	2.1	1.7	1.5	—	1.5
	F	0.7	—	—	—	0.7	1.3	1.1	0.2	0.6	0.9	1.1
France	M	1.4	1.8	0.5	0.2	0.9	2.4	2.4	2.0	1.2	0.7	1.4
	F	0.8	1.6	0.6	0.4	0.7	0.7	0.9	1.1	0.7	0.5	1.1
West Germany	M	1.2	1.9	0.6	0.3	1.1	1.3	1.8	1.5	1.4	0.9	0.6
	F	0.8	4.5	0.5	0.4	0.9	0.9	1.0	0.7	0.6	0.6	1.1
Denmark	M	0.9	3.1	0.8	—	1.3	1.5	0.8	1.8	0.4	0.5	—
	F	1.0	3.2	1.8	—	1.3	1.6	1.3	0.9	0.8	0.4	0.9
Japan	M	0.7	3.2	0.7	0.5	0.5	0.5	0.8	1.1	0.7	0.7	0.8
	F	0.5	5.0	0.7	0.3	0.3	0.3	0.4	0.5	0.6	0.6	0.9
England/Wales	M	0.7	1.4	0.7	0.3	0.8	0.8	0.7	0.8	0.8	0.3	0.5
	F	0.4	0.9	0.6	0.0	0.3	0.6	0.4	0.4	0.2	0.4	0.3

Note. A dash means no reported cases.
Sources of data: See Table 6.1.

91

of the rates for the 20 countries. Second, homicide rates among adolescents and young adults are much lower than suicide rates for most countries. The youth in the United States have the second highest homicide rates, exceeded only by Mexico; 15- to 24-year-olds in Japan have the lowest. Third, male rates are almost invariably higher than female rates for adolescent suicide and homicide (with the exception of younger female adolescent homicide rates).

As noted above, cross-cultural data can also provide information on which aspects of suicide and homicide may be culture-bound and which might be considered more culture-free or universal. For example, Tables 6.1 and 6.2 suggest that the quantity of suicides and homicides may be culture-bound, as there exists a wide range of rates for both among the various countries. On the other hand, age and sex effects appear to be universal. For virtually all countries studied, suicide and homicide increase drastically from the ages of 5–14 to 15–24. Sex effects also seem to be culture-free: Males have higher rates for suicide and homicide at nearly every age.

Suicide and homicide rates can also be combined to give an aggregate rate. Table 6.3 presents the aggregate rate for all 20 countries. Two findings are particularly noteworthy. First, again, there is a wide range of rates—from the highest of 64.1 (males) and 23.5 (females) per 100,000 population for Hungary, to the lowest of 7.0 (males) and 2.2 (females) for Greece. This range, with the highest rate being approximately 5–10 times the lowest, tends to hold for the 5–14 and 15–24 age groups as well. Second, countries with the highest aggregate rates for all ages tend also to show high rates among the younger age groups; countries with the lowest overall rates have low rates in the younger groups. That is, the rates tend to be consistent across the various age groups for each country. For 5- to 14-year-olds, the highest rates are seen in Mexico, Hungary, and the United States; for 15- to 24-year-olds, the highest rates are found in Norway, the United States, and Finland; for all ages, the highest rates are seen in Hungary and Finland. The lowest rates tend to be seen among countries such as Greece and England/

TABLE 6.3. Aggregate Suicide and Homicide Rates for 20 Countries by Age and Sex, 1990

Country		All ages	5–14 years	15–24 years
Hungary	M	64.1	3.2	21.7
	F	23.5	1.4	9.3
Finland	M	54.3	1.5	54.5
	F	14.0	—	13.8
Austria	M	36.7	0.6	26.8
	F	15.5	1.9	6.4
United States	M	36.6	2.8	54.9
	F	9.0	1.6	10.2
Mexico	M	34.6	3.4	40.5
	F	4.3	1.5	4.8
Denmark	M	33.1	1.0	15.4
	F	17.3	—	5.3
Switzerland	M	33.1	0.5	26.3
	F	14.0	1.9	7.4
France	M	31.0	0.6	15.0
	F	11.9	0.5	5.1
Czechoslovakia	M	29.6	0.8	13.5
	F	10.5	0.7	5.8
Poland	M	26.1	1.4	18.5
	F	6.3	0.7	3.3
Bulgaria	M	25.8	2.7	19.5
	F	10.3	1.3	4.8
Norway	M	25.1	1.9	55.2
	F	8.6	—	6.9
Yugoslavia	M	24.5	1.3	11.8
	F	10.3	0.7	4.2
West Germany	M	23.6	0.7	16.1
	F	10.4	0.5	5.4
Uruguay	M	23.6	1.5	19.1
	F	6.2	1.5	6.2
Canada	M	23.1	1.7	28.1
	F	6.7	1.0	6.7
Japan	M	21.1	0.9	9.7
	F	12.9	0.5	5.0
Portugal	M	16.0	0.7	9.8
	F	5.4	0.4	3.5
England/Wales	M	12.8	0.4	12.5
	F	4.1	0.0	2.3
Greece	M	7.0	0.5	6.8
	F	2.2	—	1.8

Sources of data: See Table 6.1.

Wales. The aggregate rates for the United States tend to be higher than those of most countries.

Finally, the longitudinal relationship between suicide and homicide rates deserves mention. Given the strong association between youth suicide and homicide rates in the United States, it is of interest to note whether or not a similar association is seen cross-culturally. Thus far, of six countries examined in a preliminary study, four tend to show similar trends in longitudinal youth suicide and homicide rates (Australia, Canada, England, Finland). Some of the patterns are increases in rates from the late 1960s into the mid- to late 1970s, with a subsequent leveling off or decrease in rates. Thus, it would appear that the strong association between suicide and homicide among youth is not confined to the United States.

DEMOGRAPHIC VARIABLES AND SUICIDE/HOMICIDE IN SELECTED COUNTRIES

Having examined suicide and homicide patterns in cross-cultural perspective, we now explore the relationship between demographic variables and adolescent suicide and homicide for selected countries. As described in Chapter 5, demographic variables may be related to adolescent suicide and homicide in the United States. This section investigates whether or not similar results are found in countries other than the United States. In other words, to what extent are the effects of demographic variables on suicide and homicide patterns among youth culture-bound, and to what extent might they be viewed as more universal phenomena? Two sets of data address this issue. First, cross-sectional data based on responses from thousands of adolescents in nine countries (Offer et al., 1988), as well as the results of related studies, are examined. Second, longitudinal data dealing with suicide rates and population shifts among the youth of six countries are explored.

Cross-Sectional Data

Offer and colleagues (1988) studied thousands of adolescents in 10 countries using the Offer Self-Image Questionnaire (OSIQ), a standardized structured personality test that assesses the adjustment and psychological world of youth between the ages of 13 and 19. The 10 countries were Australia, Bangladesh, Hungary, Israel, Italy, Japan, Taiwan, Turkey, the United States, and West Germany. In the study of demographic variables, all countries were used with the exception of Japan, for which data on younger age groups were not available.

Demographic variables showed significant relationships with four of the OSIQ scales. First, the higher the proportion of adolescents in a country's population, the less positive the affect reported by its teenagers. The variable "Percent of 14- to 18-year-olds in the total population" showed significant negative correlations with the OSIQ Emotional Tone scale (a measure of adolescents' emotional tone and mood) for all four age and sex groups (see Table 6.4).

Second, a high proportion of adolescents in a country's population was associated with worse social (or peer) relationships among the teenagers. Better peer relationships were related to a lower proportion of teenagers in the countries. The variable "Percent of 14- to 18-year-olds in the total population" demonstrated significantly negative correlations with the OSIQ Social Relationships scale (see Table 6.4).

Third, a high proportion of adolescents was associated with more manifest psychopathology. The variable "Percent of 14- to 18-year-olds in the total population" showed significant negative correlations with the OSIQ Psychopathology scale (a high score on the Psychopathology scale is indicative of a low incidence of such emotional symptoms as anxiety or loneliness).

Fourth, in countries where adolescents constitute a low percentage of the total labor force, teenagers reported relatively good ability to cope. Offer et al. (1988) noted that the

TABLE 6.4. Correlations between Offer Self-Image Questionnaire (OSIQ) Scales and Demographic/Economic Variables

Variable	OSIQ scale	Younger males	Older males	Younger females	Older females
1. Percent of 14- to 18-year-olds in the total population	Emotional Tone	−.79*	−.80*	−.64*	−.74*
	Social Relationships	−.84*	−.76*	−.59*	−.74*
	Psychopathology	−.76*	−.72*	−.72*	−.74*
2. Percent of 15- to 19-year-old males in the labor force	Mastery of the External World	−.83*	−.12	−.67*	−.72*
3. Gross national product (GNP)	Emotional Tone	.65*	.67*	.68*	.79*
	Social Relationships	.70*	.60*	.47	.82*
4. Per capita income	Body and Self-Image	.78*	.80*	.52	.68*
	Sexual Attitudes	.35	.58*	.75*	.87*
5. Educational expenditures per capita	Social Relationships	.63*	.64*	.52	.83*
	Psychopathology	.53	.62*	.62*	.65*

Source of data: Offer et al. (1988).

*$p < .05$ level (two-tailed test; $df = 7$).

better coping of adolescents in countries in which they form a relatively low proportion of the labor force may be a function of the adolescents' reference or comparison groups: Adolescents in the work force may be comparing themselves unfavorably to older persons already working. This finding may also be related to economic factors, in that more adolescents in the work force may indicate the existence of economic conditions unfavorable to adolescents' sense of well-being (see below).

To summarize these data, a high proportion of adolescents in a country's population is associated with adolescents' reporting poorer mood, poorer social relationships, and more psychopathology. These findings are particularly interesting in light of the data presented in Chapters 4 and 5. The population model research (Hendin, 1982; Holinger and Offer, 1981, 1982; Holinger et al., 1987) has suggested that a high proportion of adolescents in the population is associated with increased rates of youth suicide and homicide. The findings by Offer et al. (1988) in nine countries expand this relationship between demographic variables and mortality in two ways. First, the data suggest that demographic variables are related to adolescents' psychopathology and mood, in addition to mortality; second, they suggest that the relationship between demographic variables and psychopathology is not confined to the United States, but is seen in other countries and cultures as well. Furthermore, the study by Offer et al. (1988) is consistent with the findings of Klerman et al. (1985) and Easterlin (1980) regarding the impact of demography on various forms of psychopathology and social phenomena among youth, as we discuss below.

As described in Chapter 5, demographic and economic variables are closely linked: Population shifts, birth rates, and economic variables are closely interconnected. Brenner (1971, 1979) has been particularly effective in showing how economic variables (e.g., unemployment rates) can affect mortality rates. The cross-cultural data of Offer et al. (1988) also support the interaction between the economy and psychopathology among the young. Offer et al. (1988) studied a number of economic variables and related them to several OSIQ scales for thousands of adolescents in the nine countries noted above. Three economic variables correlated significantly with OSIQ scales. First, the gross national product of the countries showed positive correlations with the Emotional Tone and Social Relationships scales. Second, per capita income correlated positively with the Body and Self-Image and Sexual Attitudes scales. Third, educational expenditures per capita showed significant positive correlations with the Social Relationships and Psychopathology scales (i.e., the higher the educational expenditure, the lower the reported symptomatology; as noted above, a high score on the Psychopathology scale is indicative of a low incidence of symptoms). These results are summarized in Table 6.4. The results tend to expand Brenner's (1971, 1979) work and suggest that in a variety of countries, economic variables are associated not only with mortality but also with a wide range of psychopathology and adolescents' feelings about themselves.

Finally, two other cross-cultural studies are worth examining because they have addressed the potential impact of demographic variables with a cross-sectional study. Braungart and Braungart (1989) investigated 123 countries and determined the "youth–adult ratio" (i.e., the number of youth relative to the number of adults) for each nation. They found a wide range in this ratio among the various nations. Furthermore, the youth–adult ratio and the level of national development were found to vary together: The higher the ratio, the lower the development level. A higher youth–adult ratio was more likely to be found among younger, less democratic nations, as well as those with lower educational expenditures and secondary school enrollment.

The last study to be examined in this context is that of Stack (1988). Stack investigated "relative cohort size" (RCS)—that is, the proportion of young people (15- to 29-year-olds) to middle-aged people (30- to 64-year-olds)—and its relation to youth suicide rates for a variety of countries with different economic bases from 1950 to 1980. Thus, Stack explored the interaction between demographic and economic variables in a cross-cultural perspective. He used data from three sets of nations, categorized by their efforts to promote economic welfare for the lower classes: capitalist, welfare capitalist, and communist. The capitalist nations were Australia, Austria, Belgium, Canada, and England; the welfare capitalist countries were Denmark, Norway, and Sweden; the communist nations were Bulgaria, Czechoslovakia, Hungary, and Poland. Stack found that the RCS was usually significantly associated with suicide trends in capitalist nations, was not significantly related to suicide in the welfare capitalist set, and was equally likely to be related or unrelated to suicide in the communist group. Stack (1988) contended that the RCS declines in importance in explaining suicide as economic welfare is determined more by central planning, as opposed to supply-and-demand factors. He also suggested that in the welfare capitalist countries, economic policies such as full employment and redistributive measures may act as a buffer for the young—a cushion against the potential perils of RCS. Thus, Stack not only provided data on the relationship between demographic variables and suicide fluctuations, but provided evidence that economic conditions play a role in determining the countries in which youth suicide may be most affected by population shifts among the young.

Longitudinal Data

In addition to the cross-sectional data presented above for several countries, cross-cultural longitudinal data are also available to help address the issue of demographic variables and suicide/homicide among the young. Unfortunately, few cross-cultural studies have explored both longitudinal and demographic data. For example, a recent study of youth suicide in Finland documented longitudinal trends quite similar to those seen in the United States (increases from the 1950s to the late 1970s, with recent leveling off), but there was no mention of demographic data and the possible associations (Aro et al., 1992).

As noted in Chapter 5, in the United States several investigators have noted relationships between population shifts and suicide rates among adolescents (e.g., Solomon and Hellon, 1980; Murphy and Wetzel, 1980; Hendin, 1982; Holinger and Offer, 1981, 1982; Holinger et al., 1988). In particular, the population model studies (Hendin, 1982; Holinger and Offer, 1981, 1982; Holinger et al., 1988) have shown that increases (and decreases) in the proportion of young people in the United States are accompanied by increases (and decreases, respectively) in youth suicide rates; the opposite trend has been found for adult groups (Holinger et al., 1987). The importance of these findings lies not just in the better understanding they provide of the shifts in suicide rates, but also in the potential for the prediction of these rates.

In order to begin to study the relationships between demographic variables and suicide/homicide on a cross-cultural basis, we have examined the suicide rates for 15- to 24-year-olds and the proportion of 15- to 24-year-olds for the years 1960 through the mid-1980s, for the following six countries: Australia, Canada, Hungary, Italy, Japan, and West Germany. The results of this preliminary study are as follows. The patterns for Australia and Canada correspond most closely to those of the United States; that is, increases (and decreases) in population shifts among 15- to 24-year-olds correspond to increases (and decreases) in their suicide rates. For these two countries, this pattern reaches statistical significance. Italy shows a trend similar to that of Australia and Canada, but the trend does not reach statistical significance. The patterns for West Germany are less clear; they tend toward the U.S. pattern only for the mid-1960s to the late 1970s, without statistical significance.

The pattern for Hungary runs counter to that of the United States; that is, in Hungary the increases (and decreases) in the proportion of 15- to 24-year-olds correspond to decreases (and increases) in their suicide rates. The results for Hungary reach statistical significance. Japan shows trends similar to those of Hungary, but without consistent statistical significance.

Thus, these data suggest that the positive relationship between population shifts and suicide rates among adolescents is not confined to the United States. On the other hand, the data suggest that this relationship is by no means a universal one, as two countries show an inverse effect.

DISCUSSION

Cross-cultural data such as these aid in determining which aspects of youth suicide and homicide may be more biologic and developmental and which may be more culturally determined. Three such issues are discussed here: age, sex, and variability of rates.

With respect to age and suicide, the youngest age groups have the lowest rates for virtually all countries studied. The rates for 5- to 14-year-olds tend to be lowest, followed by those for 15- to 24-year-olds. The consistency of this finding across various cultures would seem to speak to the biologic aspects of youth suicide (the gradual emergence of major affective and thought disorders), as well as to developmental issues (cognition, onset of formal operations, etc.). It is of interest to note that in the United States the rates for 15- to 24-year-olds are not that much lower than the rates for adults—a finding that seems to indicate specific social pressures on U.S. youth. The situation for homicide is somewhat different. For most countries the highest homicide rates are found among 25- to 44-year-olds, with lower rates for 15- to 24-year-olds. For the United States, the homicide rates for 15- to 24-year-olds are as high as or higher than those for the 25- to 44-year-olds. This would suggest that in the United States various social pressures exist for the 15- to 24-year-olds that contribute to the proportionately higher homicide rates among them.

With respect to sexual differentiation, male rates are consistently higher than female rates for suicide and homicide for virtually all countries and age groups. Although socialization processes may account for some of this difference, the consistency of the male–female finding would seem to be more rooted in biologic aspects.

The variability in the rates across cultures also deserves to be mentioned. For suicide among youth, the highest and lowest rates for the various countries differ by a factor of about 10. For example, Table 6.1 shows that Finland has the highest rates (50.9 per 100,000 population for males, 11.0 for females) and Greece the lowest (5.0 and 1.2, respectively). This factor of 10 tends to hold for most age groups when the various countries are compared. However, the highest–lowest difference for youth homicide is far greater, closer to a factor of 50: for 15 to 24-year-olds, Mexico has the highest rates (35.5 for males, 3.6 for females) and Japan the lowest (0.5 and 0.3, respectively). The variability in the range of youth homicide decreases dramatically if we exclude Mexico and the United States. The massively high rates in these two countries would suggest cultural factors peculiar to the youth in those countries (i.e., serious culturally determined problems that predispose youth to homicide).

Any attempt to understand phenomena as complex as youth suicide and homicide will lead in time to an inquiry about the various degrees of biologic and cultural influence. With respect to the United States, the results of the cross-cultural data and the discussion above can be summarized as follows: The high homicide rates among youth and the proportionately high suicide rates among youth (relative to other U.S. age groups) show that specific U.S. cultural factors combine with culturally independent biologic factors to create a serious problem for this younger age group. The cultural and social pressures accounting for this situation probably include the economy and related issues of poverty and education; the size of the 15- to 24-year-old cohort; the availability of guns; and drugs.

Finally, the epidemiologic–clinical interaction is of interest. In particular, in clinical work with youth, the cross-cultural data should serve as a dramatic reminder of the high risk for older male adolescents.

CHAPTER SEVEN

Suicide: Intervention and Prevention

Most adolescents who commit suicide have diagnosable psychiatric disorders, such as a major affective disorder (bipolar disorder or major depression), schizophrenia, character disorder, or a combination of these disorders. Comorbidity of these disorders with substance abuse appears to be especially lethal. Various developmental and psychodynamic issues are discussed. Options in the treatment of suicidal youth include psychotherapy and psychoanalysis, pharmacotherapy, family therapy, and hospitalization. Summaries of major reviews dealing with prevention are presented.

ASSESSMENT AND TREATMENT

Introduction

The epidemiologic data concerning suicide are extensive. By contrast, clinical studies of the treatment of suicidal individuals are sparse and largely based on clinical reports that are not amenable to statistical interpretation. This makes the process of building a bridge between epidemiologic data and clinical practice complex. Epidemiologic data, by their nature, are related to measurable, external characteristics, pressures or stressors. As discussed earlier, these include readily identifiable personal characteristics (e.g., age, sex, and race) or social indicators (e.g., poverty, joblessness, and interrupted education). Other specific risk factors include the availability of guns in the house and concurrent substance

abuse. Furthermore, since epidemiologic data are group statistical data, their application to the understanding of the
clinical treatment of an individual case is difficult.

Clinicians generally do not rely on epidemiologic data
in assessing suicidal risk, nor do they use predictive scales.
They use clinical criteria in assessing suicidal risk. For the
individual patient, these involve internal vulnerabilities such
as genetic predisposition, character structure, and the presence of significant mental illness. Truant et al. (1991) surveyed a group of 81 Canadian psychiatrists and asked them
to rank-order, from a list of 16 factors from the literature,
the 10 most important risk factors they used in assessing a
suicidal patient. These proved to be the following: (1) degree
of hopelessness, (2) communicated ideation or plan, (3) previous attempts, (4) level of mood and affect, (5) quality of
relationships, (6) signs and symptoms of depression, (7) social integration, (8) recent loss of relationship, (9) symptoms
of mental status, and (10) willingness to accept help.

The use of rating scales to predict suicidal behavior of
an individual at risk has been explored extensively. Garrison
et al. (1991) reviewed 29 suicide assessment instruments for
adolescents and young adults . They found substantial variation in these products, depending on their intended use as
clinical or research tools. Other variation depended on the
developers' theoretical ideology, the scales' intended use, and
scale format. These questionnaires ranged in content from a
few questions to over 200 and contained 461 discrete items.
The authors were critical of several features of these scales.
Most fundamental was that little or no attention was paid
to assessing construct, predictive, or discriminant validity.
A lack of attention to validity may explain why different
researchers and clinicians, using different scales, derive in-
consistent and contradictory results. Other concerns included a lack of clarity about the intended purpose of the
instrument and a misplaced focus on assessing suicidal ideation. This latter issue is an important weakness, since the
relationship between ideation and completed suicide is as yet
unknown. Intrinsic and extrinsic factors that lead from
suicidal ideation to attempted suicide and then to completed
suicide are only speculative at this point.

This does not mean that epidemiologic data are useless in the clinical assessment of individual suicidal youth, but rather that they are not used effectively. In practice, the epidemiologic data on risk factors could be of value if researchers could identify which factors are useful in predicting high suicide risk. When epidemiologic studies show that young males are at higher risk of completed suicide than young females, the studies have identified a risk factor. Among the risk factors distinguished by epidemiologic studies are the following: Older white male adolescents and young adults are at higher risk than other adolescents; the presence of a psychiatric disorder increases the risk of suicide; concurrent drug and alcohol use are highly correlated with suicide; the presence of lethal means of suicide (especially firearms) increases the risk of death; and most completers have a history of prior attempts. Thus, a clinical evaluation of a young person with suicidal ideation should include an appreciation of these characteristics in assessing the likelihood of suicide completion. In general, the greater the number of risk factors present, the more serious the suicide risk.

However, the current state of the art for suicide prediction in an individual instance is unreliable. This is well illustrated by the study conducted by Furst and Huffine (1991). They sent out the case histories of two men who completed suicide and two who had not. Three hundred members of the American Association of Suicidology responded. The two men who completed suicide were rated by these experts as *less* vulnerable to suicide than were the two who did not. Furthermore, the suicide victims were rated lower on the vulnerability scale than would have been expected by chance.

Finally, the applicability of epidemiologic data in the treatment of suicidal youth is limited by the complex social, familial, and individual issues confronting the therapist who treats a suicidal patient. The knowledge base and skills that a successful therapist needs come from a different tradition with different challenges. However, it is important for clinicians to appreciate the value of epidemiologic research in illuminating the larger context of suicide.

Treatment of self-destructive adolescents presents

many challenges. A clinician often encounters resistance from both the patient and the family. Parental reaction can range from denial or minimizing the behavior to anxious and crippling overprotectiveness. Though they are not always willing allies in supporting treatment, parents expect the therapist to stop the self-destructive behavior. Treatment is further complicated by the significant comorbidity that accompanies suicidal acts and the complexity of the behavior that underlies suicide attempts. Finally, there is a lack of knowledge about how to insure success in treatment.

Any approach to the treatment of youth with suicidal ideation or suicide attempt behavior must begin with a competent assessment combined with a knowledge of risk factors. The importance of risk factors in the prevention of suicide has been described in earlier chapters. Clinicians are frequently challenged by the problem of assessing the seriousness of suicidal behavior in a teenager. Lacking clear guidelines, many will either underestimate or overestimate the seriousness of the suicidal thoughts or behaviors. This section focuses on approaches to assessment and treatment of the suicidal youth and his or her family.

Literature

A review of published studies on the treatment of suicidal youngsters can give a perspective on the prospects for decreasing suicide risk and preventing future suicidal episodes. The literature on the treatment of suicidal adolescents is less extensive than that dealing with other facets of suicidology, such as epidemiology, psychodynamics, or prevention. There are no controlled outcome studies of treatment of adolescent suicide attempters. This is not surprising, considering the paucity of outcome studies of any form of treatment with emotionally disturbed children and youth. The controversy and uncertainty surrounding the etiology and causes of youth suicide and suicidal behavior add to the problem of designing controlled studies. Suicide is a complex behavior that cuts across many diagnostic groups and personality types. It may have genetic as well as neuropsychiatric influences. Also, it is difficult to get a consensus about what needs to be treated in suicidal youth. Clinically, few attributes may separate suicidal adolescents from other psychologically disturbed adolescents. Brent et al. (1988) showed that virtually no characteristics differentiated between adolescent suicidal completers and hospitalized suicidal adolescents.

There is still considerable controversy about whether or not suicide and suicide attempt behavior are on a psychologic and behavioral continuum (Brent et al., 1988: Shafii et al., 1985) or are "separate but overlapping entities" (Shaffer and Bacon, 1989). The evidence from numerous psychologic autopsy studies of adolescents shows that over 90% of adolescents who complete suicide have sufficient symptoms to meet *Diagnostic and Statistical Manual of Mental Disorders,* third edition, revised (DSM-III-R) criteria for a psychiatric disorder (Brent et al., 1988; Shafii et al., 1985; Rich et al., 1986; Shaffer, 1988). Such data suggest that effective treatment of serious psychopathology could have a significant impact on youth suicide. In spite of this evidence of prevalent and severe psychopathology among suicide completers, many experts still emphasize the importance of life stresses or untenable psychosocial conditions as the cause of suicide in youth, and tailor their prevention and treatment efforts to alleviation of these conditions. This strategy may have little payoff in reducing completed suicides or repeated suicide attempts.

Trautman (1989), in his review of treatment strategies for the *Report of the Secretary's Task Force on Youth Suicide,* accurately describes the lack of scientific foundation for favoring any treatment intervention with suicidal attempters over another:

> I can state quite simply that there are no specific treatment modalities for adolescent suicide attempters. That is, there are no treatment studies—psychotherapeutic, behavioral, or psychopharmacologic—which show that a clearly defined treatment approach is superior to no treatment or to some other treatment. There are many descriptions of treat-

ment—individual, family, group, insight-oriented, behavioral, cognitive and so forth—but no evidence that
suicide attempters who are treated might not have done just
as well without that treatment. (p. 3-253)

In spite of this accurate but gloomy statement, no clinician can ignore the task of treating the individual adolescent
suicide attempter. The literature offers some clinical case
reports, but most published recommendations for treatment
of the suicidal adolescent derive from the authors' personal
biases, styles, or theoretical orientations. Where does this
leave clinicians? Certainly a nihilistic position is not very
helpful to those faced with a suicidal adolescent. What can be
recommended are standard techniques for assessment of
psychiatric and substance abuse problems, and treatment
strategies based on the clinician's understanding of the
adolescent's diagnosis, dynamics, family situation, psychosocial stressors, risk factors, and prognosis.

Suicidal Ideation and Attempts

"Suicidal ideation" refers to thinking about or fantasizing
about killing oneself. Before a suicide attempt, there are
thoughts and fantasies of suicide. Suicidal thoughts are widely prevalent and are underreported among adolescents.
Earls (1989) has reviewed some of the data from a longitudinal study of over 2,000 patients aged 13–18 in several
primary care settings over a 2-year period. The sample consisted of a majority of African-Americans (71%) and females
(77%). Since African-American females have one of the lowest reported rates of completed suicide, we might expect a
low level of reported suicidal ideation and attempt behavior.
The data did not bear this out. Of the eventual respondents,
19% thought a lot about death, 9% wanted to die, and 7%
thought about committing suicide. Two percent reported a
suicide attempt in the prior 2 years.

The Epidemiologic Catchment Area study gives data
for youth in the 18–24 age range. Of this age group sample,

23% had thoughts of death, 6% expressed a desire to die, 12% reported suicidal ideation, and 3% had made a suicide attempt in the past, although the number of years included were not specified (Mościcki et al., 1989). This may indicate that there is a significant underreporting of suicide ideation and suicide attempts in clinical settings. According to these data, almost 1 in 4 young adults reported thoughts of death, 1 in 16 expressed a desire to die, and 1 in 8 reported suicidal ideation.

Suicide Completers and Contact with Mental Health Professionals

"Suicide completion" refers to self-inflicted death. Postmortem studies of adolescents who complete suicide also indicate that they do not comprise a homogeneous group. A variable percentage of them have some contact with the mental health profession, but they rarely are in treatment at the time of the suicide. Often contact is brief, involving only an evaluation or a few supportive visits (Litman, 1989). Brent et al. (1988) found that adolescents who completed suicide differed from suicide-attempting inpatients in having a history of one or more prior contacts with a mental health professional. Sixty-six percent of the inpatients had prior contact with a mental health professional, while only 33% of completers did. Only 2 out of 27 completers in Brent et al.'s sample were in active treatment at the time of their death. Shafii et al. (1985, 1988), in their psychologic autopsy research, determined that 45% of the suicide victims had at least one prior contact with a mental health professional, but that only one of them was in active care at the time of the suicide.

Suicide Attempters and Follow-Up Care

"Suicide attempt" refers to a self-inflicted and self-destructive act or behavior that one believes will cause death, but that is unsuccessful. Generally, suicidal behavior should be considered evidence of serious psychopathology in a youth and his or her family. It also indicates the failure of usual coping mechanisms to deal with stress.

A large percentage of adolescent suicide attempters do not follow through with recommended outpatient treatment. A study by Taylor and Stansfield (1984) of 50 youths (82% female) admitted to a pediatric unit after a suicide attempt by overdose showed that 44% did not keep their scheduled outpatient appointment. Research by Litt and coworkers (1983) revealed that 61% of their sample did not comply with follow-up recommendations. A study by Viale-Val et al. (1984) of adolescents accepted for treatment at an adolescent outpatient clinic revealed that 15% of the sample presented with a complaint of suicidal behavior. These suicidal youngsters were found to drop out of treatment more often than adolescents presenting with other problems. Of the suicidal adolescents, 27% did not keep their first appointment, 53% dropped out during the initial assessment phase (three sessions), and 13% dropped out in later stages of treatment. A similar study by Trautman and Rotheram (1986, cited in Trautman, 1989) of 77 adolescents treated in an emergency room for self-injury revealed that 23% failed to keep their first appointment, 19% dropped out during the initial assessment period (one or two visits), and 27% refused treatment or dropped out of treatment after the initial assessment. This was in spite of the significant efforts made to insure compliance by telephone calls and letters following the missed appointments.

We can only speculate about why there is such a poor rate of compliance with follow-up recommendations. One answer is that the attempt has served its purpose and is followed by a period of conflict resolution and relief of stress in the family. Further treatment then has no purpose. Of course, resistance to treatment or fear of being labeled mentally ill may also play a part in this noncompliance. Some patients who fail to keep follow-up appointments or drop out of treatment may have problems that resolve themselves quickly or do not require treatment intervention. Other adolescents may fear disrupting an already tenuous family system and are content with crisis resolution. During this time the adolescents may assure their families that they will not repeat the behavior, and/or the families give in to some of the adolescents' demands. Perhaps the answer lies in the desire of families to rationalize and deny serious problems. Often a family has a problem that no one wants revealed. Resistance can be particularly strong when a parent fears or suspects that the suicidal adolescent or siblings might be removed from the family if disclosures of parental abuse arise in the therapy session. Thus, parents will not force the teen to return for an appointment. The following case illustrates such a situation.

Marci, a 16-year-old high school student, took 30 proprietary sleeping pills in a suicide attempt. She was evaluated in a general hospital emergency room and admitted for overnight observation. The psychiatric consultant who interviewed her and the family the following day responded to parental pressure, reluctantly agreeing to discharge her to the parents' care. They would not agree to hospitalization. Circumstances of the attempt that Marci (an only child) revealed to the psychiatric consultant included increased quarrels between the parents, who were close to divorce. Marci was also having trouble concentrating on her school work and was close to failing in several subjects. Recently her father had refused to buy her an automobile because of her poor school performance. A follow-up appointment was set for 3 days later. She did not keep her clinic appointment in spite of a telephone reminder.

Four months later, Marci made another attempt with a modest overdose of tricyclic antidepressants, prescribed by the family physician for inducing sleep (25 mg amitriptyline at bedtime). This time she was admitted to the psychiatric inpatient unit and stayed 7 days. On the unit she was cooperative but very guarded; she did not appear overtly depressed. The parents were now separated, and Marci was living with her father. The mother was said to be depressed and to have a serious drinking problem, so the father was the custodial parent. Her father was reluctant to come for family interviews. When he finally came, he pressured the unit physician to discharge his daughter immediately, because she was missing too much school. He promised to make Marci come for outpatient treatment.

Marci came for three outpatient visits, driving the car her father had given her following her first attempt. During the third visit she revealed that she had been sexually abused by her father for several years with her mother's knowledge, and that this was the reason for the divorce. An investigation by child protective services was unsuccessful, because the father and Marci left the city abruptly and could not be located.

Training of Clinicians in Evaluation

Adolescents with psychiatric emergencies usually present with multiple problems. Family turmoil, school problems, substance abuse, and covert psychiatric problems often make evaluation and diagnosis difficult at best. Such youth are more likely to be diagnosed as having an adjustment or conduct disorder than as having either a personality disorder or psychosis (Hillard et al., 1987). Suicidal ideation or suicide attempt behavior is common and is often missed because of an adolescent patient's obfuscation or a clinician's in-experience in evaluating suicidal behavior in adolescents.

Clinicians need education and training to be able to conduct a meaningful interview with a suicidal adolescent, to diagnose mental illness, and to develop a strategy for intervention and follow-up. The ability to assess suicidality in adolescents is a critical clinical skill that should be possessed by most practicing family physicians, pediatricians, and psychiatrists. Unfortunately, it is not. Medical schools and residency training programs offer little or no training in suicide assessment or in treatment approaches to the suicidal individual. Most psychiatric residency programs have some training on suicide, but it is minimal and most often deals with epidemiology rather than assessment or treatment issues. It rarely focuses on treatment issues with suicidal adolescents. Since psychiatric residents are a major resource in psychiatric emergency rooms, this lack of training is a serious deficit. Perhaps the recent research emphasis on defining risk factors will result in the development of a curriculum for systematic assessment of suicidal persons, especially adolescents.

Assessment of Suicidal Youth

Although a great deal of effort has been expended in trying to devise a reliable and valid screening instrument, there is no generally accepted instrument in widespread use. Yufit (1989) has described the difficulties of developing such schedules, and makes a plea for a major collaborative effort to develop a suicide screening checklist. Some screening questionnaires, even though they identify high percentages of youth with suicidal ideation and behavior, also include large numbers of youth who do not make attempts. As a result, these instruments are more useful for research purposes than for clinical situations.

In the absence of an acceptable and standardized suicide assessment checklist, there are only a few choices. One is to rely on the clinical interview. Unfortunately, the clinical interview is only as good as the interviewer, and thus is subjective. The clinical interview can be improved if the proper questions are asked. In questioning about suicidal ideation and intent, a clinician goes from the general to the specific. As answers are elicited that indicate the presence of suicidal risk factors, the clinician should become increasingly specific. Figure 7.1 presents a decision tree for the clinical assessment of suicidal youth. This decision tree forms the framework for organizing the discussion that follows.

In screening for current suicidal ideation or a definite plan, questions such as those in Table 7.1 should be asked. Positive answers to any of the questions in Table 7.1 should lead to a more thorough evaluation of the youth, to determine the presence of factors that would place the youth at greater risk. These are shown in Table 7.2. The greater the number of these risk factors that can be identified, the higher the risk of imminent suicidal behavior. This again highlights the importance of an integrated clinical and epidemiologic perspective, inasmuch as awareness of the various risk factors in Table 7.2 can be most useful in a combined assessment of potential suicidality and treatment options.

When an adolescent is identified as having any degree

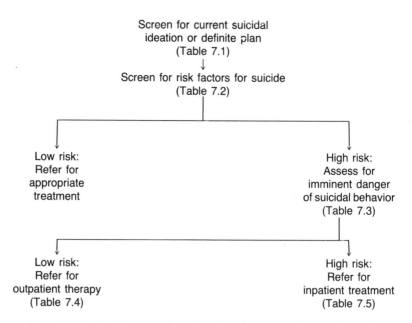

Screen for current suicidal
ideation or definite plan
(Table 7.1)
↓
Screen for risk factors for suicide
(Table 7.2)

Low risk:
Refer for
appropriate
treatment

High risk:
Assess for
imminent danger
of suicidal behavior
(Table 7.3)

Low risk:
Refer for
outpatient therapy
(Table 7.4)

High risk:
Refer for
inpatient treatment
(Table 7.5)

FIGURE 7.1. Decision tree for clinical assessment of suicidal youth.

of suicidal potential, the clinician has to make a judgment about the seriousness of the threat and the course to follow. If the present decision tree approach has been followed and low suicidal risk is identified, then the clinician can make a recommendation ranging from no follow-up to counseling or outpatient treatment. If a determination of high risk is made, then the clinician must assess the immediacy of the suicidal danger. Table 7.3 lists some of the criteria to be

TABLE 7.1. Screening Questions for Suicidal Intent

1. Has there ever been a period of 2 weeks or more when you thought a lot about death—either your own, someone else's, or death in general?
2. Has there ever been a period of 2 weeks or more when you felt like you wanted to die?
3. Have you ever thought of hurting yourself?
4. Have you ever felt so low you thought of committing suicide?
5. Do you have a plan to hurt yourself?
6. Have you ever attempted suicide?

TABLE 7.2. Risk Factors for Suicide

1. The presence of a comorbid psychiatric disorder
   a. Depressive disorder lasting more than 2 weeks, accompanied by dysphoric mood, sad, unhappy, and irritable feelings, and two or more of the following symptoms:
      1. Sleep disturbance of any kind
      2. Appetite disturbance, including either loss of appetite or over-eating
      3. Difficulty concentrating
      4. Decreased pleasure in usual activities and withdrawal from family and friends
      5. Decreased self-esteem and excessive guilt
      6. Feelings of helplessness or hopelessness
   b. Bipolar disorder with symptoms lasting a week or more or severe enough to require hospitalization; mood is elevated and expansive with irritability, and at least three of the following are present:
      1. Increased activity, restlessness, talkativeness
      2. Inflated self-esteem and grandiosity that may border on the delusional
      3. Racing thoughts and flight of ideas
      4. Decreased need for sleep, exaggerated wakefulness
      5. Distractibility
      6. Inability to recognize consequence of actions
   c. Schizophrenia symptomatology, including especially:
      1. Hallucinations
      2. Delusions
      3. Evidence of thought disorder
2. The presence of significant behavioral problems, whether or not they meet criteria for conduct disorder
   a. Problems at school, both behavioral and learning difficulties
   b. History of running away, promiscuity, reckless/dangerous driving, other risk-taking behavior
   c. Evidence of drug and alcohol abuse, including a history of missing work or school because of substance abuse, or arrests due to substance abuse
3. Family problems
   a. Documented or suspected physical or sexual abuse
   b. Psychiatric disorder in the parents, currently or by history
   c. History of completed suicide in close family members
4. Sexual identity problems, including homosexuality
5. Social isolation
   a. Inability to name friends (few close friends)
   b. Unpopularity with peers
   c. Transient personal relationships
   d. Feelings of panic and isolation when alone
6. Availability of firearms, especially in the home

TABLE 7.3. Clues to Assessing Imminent Suicidal Risk

1. Prior suicide attempts
   a. How serious were prior attempts?
   b. What was the nature of precipitating events?
   c. How lethal was the method used in previous attempts?
   d. Was prior treatment recommendation accepted or followed?
2. Nature of current suicidal ideation
   a. Is there a plan and a method for carrying out the plan?
   b. Is the method readily available?
   c. Is there significant evidence of loss of self esteem?
   d. Are there feelings of helplessness and hopelessness?
3. Nature of environmental supports
   a. Are the parents emotionally available to the youth?
   b. Are there other significant adults available to provide support?
   c. Are the parents under stress because of marital, substance abuse, physical, or mental illness problems?

Note. This table is meant to be used as a guide to clinical assessment. It is not an absolute rating scale and has not been validated for the prediction of imminent suicide.

considered in determining imminent danger of further suicidal behavior.

If this assessment yields a determination of low risk for imminent suicide, then outpatient treatment can be considered. The data on lack of follow-up for outpatient treatment of suicidal youth mandate that extra effort be expended to assure compliance with the recommendation, however. Table 7.4 lists criteria to be considered in making the decision that the suicidal youth can be managed at home.

If the suicidal threat is considered serious, the youth should be hospitalized, preferably in a psychiatric hospital with specialized adolescent services. This decision should ideally be arrived at jointly by the patient, his or her parents, and the clinician. Criteria for deciding on hospitalization are shown in Table 7.5.

Treatment Strategies

As noted earlier, many suicidal adolescents have significant comorbidity for psychiatric illness, especially affective dis-

TABLE 7.4. Criteria for Managing a Suicidal Youth at Home

1. The youth is able to control any tendencies to harm himself or herself and to call the therapist if any problems develop re: controlling suicidal impulses.
2. The parents feel able to monitor and care for the youth, and other safe conditions can be created.
3. The environment can be made safer by removing lethal means of suicide from the home. In explicit terms, this means removing guns and getting rid of or closely monitoring medications with a lethal potential. Any other agent likely to cause death must be identified and neutralized.
4. The patient and the family must agree to outpatient treatment. This is particularly critical because of the high percentage of identified suicidal youth who do not keep their first scheduled outpatient visit.

order, substance abuse, and/or conduct disorder. This pattern is not uncommon and underscores the point that treatment should be tailored to the individual. Suicidal adolescents fall into several diagnostic categories requiring differing therapeutic interventions or a combination of interventions. Among a group of suicidal youth, one may be an isolated, depressed, nonviolent youngster with a history of suicidal behavior. Another may be conduct-disordered and angry, and may have a history of substance abuse and avoidance of or hostility toward treatment interventions. A third youngster may appear to be having a "normal" adjust-

TABLE 7.5. Criteria for Hospitalization of a Suicidal Youth

1. The nature of the suicide attempt, its severity, and the presence of comorbid psychiatric conditions place the youth in the highest risk category.
2. The youth presents a clear and present danger to himself or herself if not hospitalized.
3. The parents or other caretakers are not able to provide sufficient safeguards to prevent a recurrence of the suicidal behavior.
4. In the current situation, there are not therapeutic interventions or alternative programs that can meet the patient's needs. This is essentially a risk–benefit analysis of the options of managing the adolescent in or out of the hospital.

ment reaction, with features of anxiety, perfectionistic tendencies, and narcissistic vulnerability. Brent et al. (1988) have identified bipolar affective illness as a comorbid disorder of which clinicians should be especially aware because of its increased lethality. They make the point that bipolar disorder is often undiagnosed because of the presence of conduct disorder and substance abuse problems. Treatment of such youth may require detoxification, treatment of substance abuse, lithium or other antimanic drug treatment, and psychotherapy. When we consider just these few scenarios out of many, it should be apparent that no one treatment approach fits all. Many modalities of treatment have their place in the therapy of suicidal youth, on both outpatient and inpatient bases.

Hospitalization of the Suicidal Adolescent

Hospitalization of the suicidal adolescent may be life-saving, but the clinician must be prepared for resistance from both adolescent and family. The suicidal adolescent, already suffering from low self-esteem and a sense of failure, may vigorously protest the decision to hospitalize him or her. Parents often view the decision as a reflection of their failure to communicate with or take care of their child. Many issues may be raised to argue against hospitalization: the possible stigmatization of the youngster at school or among his or her peers; the fear of the youth's being labeled as "mentally ill"; concerns about treatments to which he or she will be subjected; and fear of having him or her exposed to other mentally disturbed patients. Notwithstanding these resistances and fears, hospitalization is often the wisest course, especially when there is significant comorbidity with diagnosed mental illness or substance abuse.

Hospitalization of the suicidal youth creates a safe haven that takes pressure off both the youth and his or her parents. It affords an opportunity to do a thorough psychologic and medical evaluation. A comprehensive medical, social, and family history can be obtained. Psychologic tests and other assessment tools can be employed to gain a better understanding of the youngster. A complete physical examination with relevant laboratory examinations can be carried out, and an assessment of educational attainment and future needs can be accomplished.

The goals of hospitalization should be discussed with the adolescent and the family early in the treatment. These goals should be as clear and practical as possible. If the adolescent and parents are cooperative, it is desirable to develop these goals conjointly. For the suicidal youngster, an obvious goal is protection from self-destructive urges. When another condition such as depression or substance abuse is present, a goal can be to treat the depression with appropriate antidepressants or the substance abuse with detoxification and group or individual therapy. For conduct-disordered patients, a structured milieu and a cognitive–behavioral program can help to alter maladaptive behavioral patterns. Ultimately, the goal is to alleviate the suicidal ideation or drive and to reduce tensions or problems with the family so that the youth can be discharged.

A variety of therapeutic approaches and modalities are usually available in an adolescent inpatient psychiatric setting. Such a variety makes it possible for the staff to develop an individualized treatment plan for each adolescent. This plan should address the youth's medical, psychologic, and educational needs. Attention also must be paid to the recreational and activity needs of adolescents while in the hospital. In managing suicidal adolescents in inpatient settings, it is important to have a clear suicide precautions protocol that is known to all staff members and regularly reviewed. Newly employed staff members must be oriented to the problems of dealing with suicidal youth and must be trained in suicide precautions.

A typical multimodal inpatient unit for adolescents, including those with suicidal behaviors, should include the following formal interventions:

1. Milieu therapy with behavioral reinforcements. Milieu therapy requires a cohesive staff providing consistent verbal feedback and reinforcement to individual adolescents. The behavioral reinforcements can be based on a point sys-

tem, with points being awarded for appropriate behavior and taken away for inappropriate behavior. Privilege level is based on points earned and on the team's assessment of each adolescent's ability to handle increased privileges.

2. Individual psychotherapy provided by a trained and skilled adolescent psychotherapist.

3. Psychopharmacology for indicated and diagnosed conditions, prescribed by the treating physician with informed consent of both the adolescent and his or her parents.

4. Group psychotherapy—both large milieu groups focused on issues pertaining to congregate living and staff–patient interactions, and smaller groups dealing with individual problems such as low self-esteem and depression.

5. Family therapy, both with the adolescent and family together and with the family members separately. Parents may need their own separate treatment outside of the contract involving the patient. Psychoeducational approaches to parental effectiveness, management of suicidal behavior, and understanding of mental disorders can be included within conjoint family groups.

6. Educational programs aimed at meeting an adolescent's needs to continue in school and maintain or improve educational achievement. Special education teachers, in consultation with the therapeutic team, should develop an individualized educational plan for each youth. A behavioral reinforcement approach can make the school experience an integral part of the treatment program.

7. Activity therapy, such as exercise, excursions to parks and museums, and arts and crafts, to provide physical activity. Such therapy can also help in structuring activities of daily living and other social skills for the adolescent.

Discharge Planning.   Plans and options for discharge should be thought out and discussed well in advance of the actual discharge date. The discharge plan needs to include (1) follow-up psychiatric treatment and any necessary medical care; (2) posthospital living arrangements; (3) arrangements for continued educational or vocational needs; and (4) counseling or treatment for other family members when indicated. Before and after discharge, the adolescent should be encouraged to discuss his or her reaction to the separations from the staff, the hospital, and other patients.

Inpatient Suicide of an Adolescent. The suicide of a youngster while on an inpatient unit occurs occasionally; when it does, it has profound effects on other youngsters, the staff of the unit, and the parents. An inpatient suicide must be reviewed carefully to determine the circumstances of the suicide and what can be done to eliminate the possibility of future suicides. In addition to this review, it is important to work with the other youngsters, the unit staff, and the family. It is common for inpatient adolescents to feel some responsibility for not preventing the death of their fellow patient. They are often angry at staff members for not preventing the suicide, and harbor concerns that the staff will not be able to protect them against their own unacceptable impulses. Adolescents also need guidance with the grieving process. The staff members need considerable support, both individually and in groups. Feelings of failure and guilt, fear of being blamed, and worries about being sued for malpractice are all common reactions that need to be worked through. Parents need support with their grief and reassurance that they have done all that they could for their youngster. Parents are often angry and blame the hospital and staff for not preventing the suicide. Threats of legal action are common. Often the sensitivity with which the parents are helped and supported through the grieving process is crucial to shaping the parents' feelings about what happened.

While an inpatient on a 15-bed acute adolescent treatment unit, Tony, a 15-year-old, hanged himself with strips torn from his pajamas. He had been admitted following a suicide attempt involving carbon monoxide poisoning with his mother's automobile. His father had died of cancer about 2 years before his admission. He had not grieved for his father's death, according to his mother and older sister; however, his school work suffered, he became "difficult," and his mother suspected that he was drinking a lot of alcohol. She had difficulty disciplining him, and was angry and hurt that Tony did not approve of the man she had recently started dating.

Tony was on the inpatient unit for 2 months before his suicide. His involvement in ward activities was marginal, and he was socially isolated from other youngsters and the staff. He lost weight and began having nightmares and trouble sleeping. A diagnosis of major depression was made, and he was placed on a tricyclic antidepressant 3 weeks before the suicide occurred. He showed some slight improvement in mood and a better sleep pattern. He had no major rule infractions, and the treatment team agreed to advance him from high-risk suicide precautions to low-risk status. On low-risk status, staff members were required to know where he was at all times, and he had to be visually checked every 5 minutes.

On the evening of the suicide, Tony told the staff nurse that he was going to the bathroom. The milieu staff then became busy admitting a new, highly disruptive youngster. One staff member was sent to another unit to get a set of leather restraints. Placing the new youngster in restraints was a struggle and required assistance from another unit. Approximately 12 minutes elapsed between Tony's going to the bathroom and a staff member's walking in to find him strangled by the twisted cloth rope tied to a loose bolt on a shower stall. Resuscitation was partially successful, and he was transferred to the medical intensive care unit (MICU). Over the next 24 hours, however, it became apparent that he was brain-dead, and further heroic attempts were abandoned.

The unit psychiatrist and some daytime staff members came into the hospital that evening and held a milieu meeting to discuss the suicide. The focus was on helping the mother accept that a tragedy had occurred and helping her express sad and angry feelings. Two teen inpatients asked for individual attention, and both confided to the therapist that Tony had told them he was going to kill himself soon. They had dismissed the threat because he was always talking about suicide. Now they felt guilty because they had not alerted the staff. They were also upset that the staff had reduced his suicide precautions. Both were given special support over the next few days. The unit psychiatrist and social worker met with Tony's mother and sister at the MICU and provided supportive therapy. After Tony died, his mother gave permission for his organs to be used for transplant purposes; she expressed the wish that some good should come from his death. Staff members on duty were given an opportunity to express their feelings and given support as well.

Therapist and Treatment Staff Burnout. The treatment of chronically suicidal patients is arduous and can elicit strong countertransference reactions in the therapist and in other members of a treatment team. It is important to have clear guidelines about suicide precautions and treatment goals. Burnout is a common experience among inpatient treatment staff members who have to deal with several suicidal adolescents at the same time. For this reason, many inpatient units have an unwritten rule to limit the number of suicidal inpatients to no more than two at the same time. Among the ways to prevent burnout is to share the burden with others as much as possible. Periodic consultations with a respected colleague or regular supervision can be especially helpful.

Psychotherapy and Psychoanalysis

The lack of literature about the treatment of depressed or suicidal youth is particularly acute in regard to psychotherapy. There are few studies comparing the effectiveness of different psychotherapeutic approaches for suicidal youth, or, for that matter, examining adolescent psychotherapy in general. A meta-analysis of the effectiveness of psychotherapy with children was published by Weisz et al. (1987). It showed that the results for psychotherapy with children and adolescents were roughly similar to those found among adults; that is, 70%–80% improved. Behavioral and cognitive interventions were overrepresented in this meta-analysis, however. Most of the psychotherapeutic literature, including psychoanalytic papers, deals with single, in-depth case studies. Novick's (1984) work represents a notable exception to this tendency in the literature, as his group synthesized the results of the psychoanalyses of seven suicidal adolescents (see below).

Obviously, what any therapist brings to the treatment relationship is based on his or her training, experience, and theoretical orientation. With the current emphasis on treatments aimed at specific issues, and the limitations placed by many third-party payers on reimbursement and length of stay, there has been more interest in active and direct treatment approaches. This is consistent with the episodic nature of many adolescent problems, including suicidal behavior.

Rutter (1986) has presented some goals for psychotherapy that seem particularly appropriate for suicidal adolescents. The first of these is symptom reduction and alleviation of distress. This focuses attention on depression, conduct disorder, substance abuse, anxiety, or other symptoms that are often found in suicidal patients. A second goal is to reduce maladaptive behaviors that can impede the youngster's return to his or her family, school, or normal activities. Since many suicidal youngsters have major self-image problems and suffer from repeated failures, another goal is to encourage self-reliant behaviors. Finally, the importance of the adolescent's self-understanding—of feelings, behaviors, conflicts, relationships, and so on—cannot be overestimated. The ultimate goal is to assist the teenager to acquire the necessary skills, experiences, and self-understanding that will be useful in achieving and sustaining normative development. Psychotherapeutic interventions can be targeted to any one or to a combination of these foci.

The treatment of the suicidal adolescent is a rocky road, with many obstacles being placed in the way. The adolescent patient often gives mixed clues about what is going on, based on his or her fluctuating moods. In talking with a adolescent patient about a suicide attempt, a therapist should be direct, exploratory, and supportive—not judgmental. Since the adolescent knows what he or she did, and the therapist does not, nothing is gained from oblique inquiry or euphemistic phrases. Inquiry can help the young person identify the feelings that accompanied the suicide attempt and that may affect other daily behavior. It is important to be able to help the teenager recognize that how he or she feels is related to both past and current events. Transference and countertransference concepts can be especially useful in working with suicidal adolescents. If a patient feels inhibited about expressing feelings (especially angry ones), this should be identified as a potential cause for depression and lack of enjoyment, and the various intrapsychic, transference, and countertransference issues will need exploration. The therapist should recognize that the young person probably has deficient self-regulatory capacities, and berating the youngster for being stupid about trying to end his or her life will further diminish self-esteem and self-worth.

Hurry (1977, 1978), Novick (1984), and Hendin (1991a) are among those who have explored in some depth the psychodynamic issues and psychotherapeutic and psychoanalytic treatments of suicidal adolescents. The following two cases (summarized from the literature) provide a picture of the type of in-depth psychoanalytic work that can take place with suicidal adolescents.

Hurry (1977, 1978) presented the case of a patient named Jessie, who was seen in analysis for about 6 years from 15 to 21 years of age. Jessie had threatened to kill herself from latency onward, and she viewed herself as almost totally worthless: dirty, broken, and vicious; stupid, bad, and mad.

Jessie was the youngest daughter in a highly disturbed family. Her mother had been hospitalized for nervous breakdowns and was intensely hypochondriacal. Toward Jessie, she was perceived as being intrusive, controlling, guilt-provoking, and infantilizing. In treatment Jessie gradually expressed her awareness that her mother could not perceive her except in terms of her own needs, could not allow her to have feelings of her own. In addition, she showed marked hostility to Jessie.

Jessie's first session was delayed because an uncle had died the night before. During the first session, Jessie talked about her depression but not her suicidal feelings. The analyst told Jessie that she thought Jessie did need help, but also told her that the decision had to be Jessie's own. The analyst felt in retrospect that the latter stance was a mistake, because Jessie construed it as a total rejection. That night Jessie got into an argument, first with her boyfriend and then with an aunt. The parents joined in, shouting how wicked Jessie was, and hitting her "all over." Jessie then took 20 or 30 of her mother's pills and told a cousin, who told her not to be stupid. Her aunt also was reported to have said, "Don't take any notice of her, she's just a stupid girl." Jessie then took another 40 or 50 pills, became unconscious, and was hospitalized. She remained in a coma for 48 hours.

Hurry described Jessie's treatment by listing several dynamic factors that appeared to be behind the suicide attempt and that were worked through in the analysis. These included the wish for care and protection; defenses against the fear of abandonment (suicide appeared to be a more effective way of leaving before she could be left, an attempt to insure the object's grief, and at times an active way of abolishing pain); the wish for narcissistic union; the need to be a separate, independent person; defenses against aggression; the expression of aggression; a response to parental aggression; the expression of sexuality; defenses against sexuality; and the restoration of self-esteem (suicide had represented for Jessie a way of becoming what otherwise she had felt she could never be—phallic, competent, and successful). Hurry (1977, 1978) summarized by emphasizing that the suicide behavior in Jessie's case was highly overdetermined.

The second patient, Mary, had just turned 18 when she began her analysis. The length of the analysis in the report was 3 years, and it was implied that the analysis was continuing (Novick, 1984).

Mary was the younger of two children, having a brother 3 years older. Mary was seen as a high achiever and as well behaved, whereas her brother had always rebelled and failed at school. Mary's mother was described as "weird"; she was barely able to conceal her hostility toward her daughter, and unable to tolerate the slightest sign of hostility toward herself. The father was a college-educated, professional man who tended to deny Mary's pathology. Mary described herself as "feeling bad" for at least 4 years, and as having been preoccupied by thoughts of death and dying for many years.

Mary's suicide attempt occurred about a week after her 18th birthday and prior to her entering treatment. She drove her car down a steep embankment; the car was completely destroyed, and Mary suffered severe internal injuries and nearly died. After recovering from major surgery, she told her psychiatrist that she had intended to kill herself. Novick (1984) noted that it was only after much analysis that an understanding of the suicide attempt was achieved. He emphasized that the attempt was not an impulsive act, but the endpoint of a pathologic regression.

Mary's case is used by Novick as an example of a sequence of regression seen in several suicidal adolescents; this sequence is described in more detail below in connection with Novick's "focal research." However, mention should be made of Novick's particular stress on Mary's difficulty with separation–individuation. He stated that Mary was unable to take steps away from her mother, and that during the course of treatment she was "feeling bad" (Mary's term for unarticulated general dysphoria) as she began to see her mother as "weird." Her father and analyst then became the "bad guys," and she became more dependent on her mother and highly suicidal. The theme of protecting her mother and denying the mother's psychopathology was an important one, Novick contended. During the course of analysis, Mary recalled a forgotten incident in which she and her brother and her father were brought closer together, to the exclusion of her mother. Oedipal as well as separation–individuation issues were described as being worked through in the analysis.

In addition to the case described above, Novick's (1984) group provided extensive data on the psychoanalysis of six other suicidal adolescents. The patients were in subsidized, five-times-per-week psychoanalysis; they were nonpsychotic adolescents who had made medically serious attempts. They consisted of three females and four males, with an age range of 14–19 years.

Novick used the term "focal research" to describe the methodology of the research group. Each analyst wrote weekly reports, and all analysts met weekly as a group for 2 hours to discuss the cases. In addition, the analysts worked in pairs on each patient, each separately abstracting the other's case with specific reference to suicide (either the preceding attempt or references to suicidal thoughts and plans). Novick also noted other measures of internal reliability used by the group.

The focal research provided two sets of data: (1) information about the patients' suicidal thoughts (including memories of the actual attempts, attitudes and fantasies about suicide, etc.), and (2) the context in which these thoughts emerged. In all seven cases, suicidal thoughts were found to emerge in relation to (1) fear or feeling of abandonment; (2) fear or wish for engulfment; and (3) fear of guilt over what were felt to be omnipotent aggressive wishes toward the patients' mothers.

Perhaps most importantly, the group found evidence in each case for a step-like suicide sequence. As noted above in regard to Mary, the suicide attempt in each of the cases was not a sudden act, but the endpoint of a pathologic regression. It usually took much of the analysis to uncover this material regarding the attempt. Novick detailed 13 steps in the suicide sequence, and these are briefly outlined here.

1. For a considerable period prior to the attempt, each adolescent felt depressed and sexually abnormal, and had suicidal thoughts.

2. The adolescent attempted to take a step that represented breaking ties with the mother.

3. In each case, this attempt failed.

4. The adolescent was thrown back onto an intense infantile relationship with the mother.

5. In this state of dependency, there was anxiety resulting from sexual and aggressive preoccupations, and there was evidence that the adolescent had some awareness of the incestuous nature of his or her fantasies.

6. There was another attempt to break away from the mother, this time by appealing to another person, with the appeal taking the form of a suicide threat.

7. There was a breakthrough of aggression toward the mother, with guilt and fear of a loss of control of impulses.

8. A sense of intense panic and deadlock ensued, with suicide seen as a positive solution.

9. The adolescent turned to the external world, provoking rejection from a person other than the mother, leading to a decrease in guilt; with guilt no longer an inhibiting factor, the suicide plan was put into motion.

10. The adolescent viewed the suicide attempt as having multiple results (e.g., the world would be sorry for mistreating him or her).

11. The actual suicide attempt was made; it represented an altered ego state, a psychotic state, and a total denial of death, as well as a state of peace in which the adolescent was at one with the mother.

12. The method itself often had specific dynamic significance.

13. The adolescent felt a relief of tension and sense of calm.

Two recent clinical advances in the psychotherapy and psychoanalysis of suicidal adolescents should also be noted: the impact of infant research and developmental psychology; and advances in clinical theory and the enhanced understanding of narcissistic pathology. These two areas have made severe character disorders (e.g., so-called borderline and narcissistic personality disorders) and dyadic pathology much more understandable and treatable. With respect to infant research and developmental psychology, the work of researchers and clinicians such as Spitz, Mahler, Bowlby, Emde, Lichtenberg, Stern, and others has led to an increasingly sophisticated view of development, with important clinical implications. For example, Tomkins (1962–1963) identified eight basic affects and their facial expressions that are present at birth or shortly thereafter, each with a range from mild to intense expression: surprise–startle, interest–excitement, enjoyment–joy, distress–anguish, contempt–disgust, anger–rage, fear–terror, and shame–humiliation. Basch (1988) has suggested two others: understimulation–boredom, and sadness. Stern (1985) has described five domains of relatedness with corresponding senses of self: emergent (about 0–2 months; involves early organization and rhythms); core (about 2–7 months; involves an increasing sense of volition and consequences as a product of self-agency, self-coherence, self-affectivity, and self-history); intersubjective (about 7–18 months; includes the capacities for sharing of joint attention, intentions, and affective states [affect attunement]); verbal (about 18 months to 2.5–3.5 years; involves acquisition of language and self-reflection); and narrative (from about 2.5–3.5 years on; involves sharing of one's private representational world). This increased understanding of affects and development has led not only to better identification of the level of psychopathology and nature of developmental problems, but also to more effective treatment through the appropriate utilization of interpretive and noninterpretive interventions (Basch, 1988; Holinger, 1990b).

The second advance has resulted from additions to clinical theory and a better understanding and treatment of narcissistic pathology. Pine (1990) has suggested that psychologic data can be conceptualized as belonging in four theoretical systems: drive theory, ego psychology, object relations theory, and self psychology. The psychologies of drive, ego, and object relations have informed clinical work for many decades, but self psychology is a fairly recent addition. Suicidal adolescents are often beset by severe tension regulation problems, difficulties in self-esteem modulation, and other manifestations of dyadic pathology. Drug use, delinquent actions, and risk-taking behaviors are only a few of the potential manifestations of this type of pathology. Kernberg (1975) and Kohut (1971, 1984) are among those who have enhanced clinicians' understanding of the feelings (self-esteem difficulties, grandiosity, rage, etc.) and resultant behaviors of those suicidal adolescents with severe narcissistic pathology. In addition, self psychology has contributed specific concepts that are of use in working with many patients, including suicidal adolescents. Examples include the construct of selfobject functions (i.e., the extent to which the subject needs certain psychologic functions provided by the object in order to maintain self-cohesion and esteem) and the various selfobject transferences (mirror, idealizing, twinship). These can be quite helpful in understanding various aspects of the pathology and treatment of disturbed adolescents (Basch, 1988; Kohut, 1984).

Cognitive–behavioral therapy, aimed at correcting major reality distortions, can also be a useful psychotherapeutic approach. It is based on social learning theory and emphasizes the interrelationship among behavior, environmental events, and internal thoughts and feelings. The interventions are directed toward changing maladaptive patterns of behavior. In practice, the approach is to define the maladaptive behaviors and encourage the adolescent to keep track of the number of times and ways in which such behaviors are begun and continued. Goals for change are defined in small incremental steps, so that no one task seems insurmountable. There is extensive use of contracting to help sustain the youth between sessions. As goals are achieved, positive feedback enables the youth to feel a sense of self-mastery and self-esteem.

Cognitive–behavioral therapy is also useful in treating the excessively self-critical attitudes found in some suicidal adolescents. The techniques are the same: self-monitoring; identification of negative images, thoughts, and feelings; learning how to control these critical attitudes; and exercises to practice newly acquired skills. Of most importance are exercises designed to enhance self-esteem and reinforce positive accomplishments. Unrealistic expectations need to be worked through and put in perspective. Adolescent suicide attempters need to learn that making mistakes can be a learning experience rather than a sign of inadequacy or failure.

A number of phenomena seen in therapy of adolescent suicide attempters may mitigate against success in treatment. Some adolescents recover rapidly after a suicide attempt and deny that anything has happened. They quickly leave treatment and can rarely be engaged in psychotherapy. Other adolescents will avoid entering a treatment relationship by confiding in their peers. The result is that they withhold information from the therapist or others trying to understand and help them. It often comes as a shock to the therapist working with adolescents to discover that there is not instant trust leading to confidences. Some of these are transference issues. Adolescents may see the therapist as aloof and distant, hostile, or cold, depending on their introjects; this often parallels their view of other significant adults, such as their parents or teachers. Many suicidal adolescents appear to avoid getting involved in a therapeutic relationship because of fear of abandonment or rejection. Particularly in short-term focused therapy, great sensitivity is needed in dealing with separations or termination of therapy.

Family Therapy

Family therapy has been a mainstay in the treatment of adolescents. Many problems affecting a high-risk youngster are rooted in family conflicts. The family will bear the brunt of dealing with the adolescent as long as he or she is in the home. For these reasons, an attempt to involve the family is imperative. There are a number of schools of family treatment. These include family systems therapy, strategic family therapy, structural family therapy, conjoint family groups, psychodynamic and supportive family therapy, and psychoeducation. The choice of an approach depends upon the therapist's knowledge of techniques and skill in a particular modality. It is important that the family not be scapegoated. It is often tempting, particularly with an adolescent suicide attempter, to blame the family for the adolescent's problems; this is counterproductive, for the most part. It tends to relieve the adolescent of any responsibility for his or her own behavior, and generally alienates the family members and decreases their cooperation. Of course, with some families (such as those in which a member has sexually or physically abused a youngster), it may not be possible to do family therapy for legal or custodial reasons.

The prescription for family therapy is based upon an evaluation of the family that suggests that this approach will be useful. Like all therapy, it should have a goal. The goals can be as opposite as returning the adolescent to the family or removing him or her from the family. Often significant time and better understanding of family dynamics are needed before these goals can be finalized. It is always desirable in family therapy, as in individual therapy, to be flexible and to reassess goals as family interactions and dynamics are better understood. The clearer the goals are to the family and the youngster, the more likely they are to succeed. Even when the family accepts family therapy, it is often with reluctance and with conflicted feelings. Parents may deny or minimize the severity of the suicidal behavior (e.g., "It was just a bid for attention") for many reasons, including rationalizing the lack of need for family therapy. It is necessary to be firm with parents about the need for treatment and for their participation and support in the treatment process. For some families, a psychoeducational approach will help them understand the realistic risks of future self-destructive behavior and how to diminish them. For example, it is often difficult to get parents to remove guns or other lethal instruments from the house until they fully understand the risk to the youngster of the continued availability of these instruments, as in the following case.

Wendell was a 17-year-old white youth admitted to an inpatient service after an attempt to hang himself. He was an only child. He was depressed, had severe problems in school in spite of being a B+ student, and had several recent arrests for alcohol-related behavior. Family interviews revealed that Wendell's father and mother had been talking about a separation after 25 years of marriage. The father was a hard-drinking, successful contractor who liked to fish and hunt. He was disappointed that Wendell did not share these interests. In one family session when Wendell explained that he didn't like killing things, his father retorted, "Then why in hell did you try to kill yourself?" Wendell could not answer and remained silent through much of the rest of the session. The mother seemed to be more allied with Wendell on this issue and was proud of Wendell's ability to write well; she hoped for a journalistic or other literary career for her son. This was only one of many disagreements between the parents about Wendell's future.

After Wendell had been in the hospital for 6 weeks, a weekend pass was arranged. Before the pass, a family session dealt with the need to make sure that the house was suicide-proofed. Particular mention was made of the father's large collection of rifles and pistols, as well as of pills. It was also agreed that Wendell would not be permitted to drive alone. During the weekend, Wendell managed to open the locked cabinet holding the guns; he was looking for ammunition when his mother walked into the room. He was returned to the hospital immediately. At the next family session, the father admitted that he had not taken the warning about the guns seriously, because "the kid has been around guns all his life and never threatened to use one on himself before." The father had the weapons removed from his house to his business and bought a special gun safe to store them.

Another goal for family therapy can be to encourage parents to seek therapy for themselves. If the parents have serious problems (such as mental illness, substance abuse, ongoing marital conflict, abusive behaviors, or correctable social problems), then attempts should be made to engage them in an appropriate therapeutic endeavor. This can include group or individual therapy, participation in a self-help group for substance abusers, or referral to social agencies for evaluation and services.

Pharmacotherapy of Specific Disorders

Two recent reviews of the use of psychotropic medications with children and adolescents have pointed out the scarcity of scientific studies of the efficacy of drug treatments in these age groups (Campbell and Spencer, 1988; Rifkin et al., 1986). Most studies are open clinical trials. There are few double-blind studies of drug treatment involving children and adolescents, and results are often confusing and ambiguous. Poor study design, lack of rigor in the use of diagnostic criteria, an inadequate treatment period, and small sample size all contribute to the problem. There is a general clinical assumption that antipsychotics, antimanics, and antidepressants should be as effective in young people with diagnosed disorders as they are in adults. As Rifkin et al. (1986) note, "measurements of neurotransmitters, their metabolites, and related enzymes in blood, urine, and spinal fluid suggests that the most marked developmental changes occur at this time [i.e., adolescence]." The differences are greater for younger adolescents; however, the clinician faced with the need to treat a suicidal adolescent with a definite comorbid diagnosis of major depression, bipolar disorder, schizophrenia, panic disorder, or other condition may have no choice except to initiate psychotropic drug treatment.

Guidelines should include a diagnosis of major mental illness meeting DSM-III-R criteria; a lack of progress with other treatment modalities; a deteriorating clinical condition; and serious suicide risk. Early and effective treatment of major mental illness may prevent or ameliorate serious self-destructive behavior. Pharmacotherapy needs to be tailored to the specific diagnosed disorder. Clinical experience suggests that the clinician should not rely solely on medications; concomitant treatment with group, family, individual, and adjunctive modalities is always indicated. The recommendations that follow are general, and specifics of treatment should always be reviewed for each individual patient.

Major Depression. The relationship between suicidal ideation and depression has been widely documented for both adult and adolescent suicidal individuals. Depression should be diagnosed in suicidal adolescents by criteria similar to those used for adults. Considering the difficulties of diagnosing depression in adolescents, it is important to adhere to DSM-III-R criteria when making a decision to treat with antidepressants. That is, suicidal ideation alone should not be an indication for the use of antidepressants, but major depression that meets DSM-III-R criteria is. The presence of comorbidity for substance abuse is a factor indicating particularly high risk, especially in young men.

Imipramine and amitriptyline are probably the drugs of choice, because there has been more clinical experience with these (Ryan, 1990). The dosages should be adjusted toward the conservative side, since the dose–response curve may be different in adolescents. Dosage of imipramine should start in the range of 1.0–1.5 mg/kg/day, and should be increased by 1.0–1.5 mg/kg/day every third day until a therapeutic level is reached. The Food and Drug Administration (FDA) suggests that the daily dose not exceed 5.0 mg/kg/day for the treatment of depression in children and young adolescents. Use of second-generation tricyclics, such as desipramine and nortriptyline, is acceptable in appropriately adjusted doses.

Before initiating treatment with tricyclics, a physician should obtain an electrocardiogram (EKG); routine blood and urine tests; thyroid function tests; and tests of blood urea nitrogen, serum creatinine, and electrolytes. During treatment it is advisable to monitor the plasma level of tricyclics, for several reasons. Plasma levels enable the physician to determine that the medication is being taken and that a therapeutic level has been attained. Plasma level monitoring can also prevent cardiotoxicity and neurotoxicity. EKG monitoring until the patient is on a therapeutic level can be helpful in detecting early signs of cardiotoxicity as well. Lithium can be considered for the treatment of depression in adolescents, particularly in those who do not respond to tricyclics or whose symptoms include aggressive and impulsive disorders; a discussion of lithium carbonate follows this section. The response rate to antidepressant use in adolescents is generally lower than in adults.

Using tricyclics on an outpatient basis with adolescents requires considerable cooperation for the family and the patient. The number of pills dispensed at any one time should not exceed 50% of the lethal dose unless parents can guarantee a secure, locked repository for the medication and control over dispensing. These drugs are potentially lethal, as any emergency room physician will attest. They require careful monitoring on the part of parents or other adults to prevent a fatal overdose. Parents should also be instructed to observe for common side effects.

Bipolar Disorder. Bipolar disorder in adolescents often presents as depression or is mistaken for schizophreniform disorder. Bipolar youngsters are at special risk for suicide (Kovacs and Puig-Antich, 1989); therefore, eliminating or ameliorating the severity of future episodes of bipolar disorder has potential preventive value. The earlier the onset of the disease, the greater the risk for repeated suicide attempts.

Bipolar disorder should be treated with appropriate medication, usually lithium carbonate. Before lithium is prescribed for adolescents, contraindications should be ruled out. These are similar to those for adults and include kidney and heart disorders, chronic diarrhea, and use of diuretics. The laboratory workup should include sodium and potassium levels, blood urea nitrogen levels, creatinine clearance, and thyroid function studies. Although the pharmacokinetics of lithium in adolescents are not well worked out, it is wise to base doses on body weight. Lithium levels should be monitored to be maintained between 0.7 and 1.4 mEq/liter. Levels must be determined 12 hours after the last dose. It takes approximately 4 days to achieve a steady state after change in dosage. Dosages may have to be increased in youngsters with efficient renal clearance of lithium. In adolescent girls, one must consider the likelihood of pregnancy before prescribing lithium. Side effects of lithium use with adolescents include weight gain, decreased motor activity, sedation, gastrointestinal distress, polyuria, and headache. Other complications may include hypothyroidism, as well as deposition of lithium in bone, which may inhibit growth. Lithium is less sedating than neuroleptics, and adolescents generally tolerate it well (Campbell et al., 1984).

Carbamazepine and other anticonvulsant medications have been used for treatment-resistant bipolar disorders in adults, with some success. Their use in adolescents is less well documented in the literature. The physician prescribing these should be aware of FDA requirements for prescribing a drug not approved for a particular condition.

Schizophrenia and Other Psychotic Disorders. Schizophreniform psychosis, schizophrenia, and other psychoses of suicidal adolescents should be treated with appropriate antipsychotic medication. Differential diagnosis is important, since several drugs of abuse can cause symptoms that resemble schizophreniform psychosis. In these cases, waiting several days can result in complete clearing of the psychotic symptoms and the suicidal behavior. High-potency neuroleptics such as haloperidol have wide clinical use, probably because they are less sedating at therapeutic doses. A complete blood count and a liver profile should be obtained before initiating treatment and at regular intervals during treatment. Side effects can be treated with antiparkinsonian agents. Dysphoria induced by medication is a major factor in noncompliance. Due to the problem of dyskinesia, it is important to keep doses at the minimal effective level and to keep length of treatment as brief as clinically

possible. Lithium has also been used to treat chronic psychoses of adolescents, with some success.

Treatment of Substance Abuse and Suicidality

Increased risk of suicide is associated with substance abuse in
both adolescents and adults. Fowler et al. (1986), in their
study of suicide in San Diego, found that 58% of completed
suicides were associated with drug abuse; of these, 40% met
the criteria for a principal diagnosis of substance abuse. The
Epidemiologic Catchment Area Study (Robins et al., 1984)
reported an 11%–18% lifetime prevalence for substance
abuse. Thus, suicidal adolescents with a history of substance
abuse should be assumed to be at very high risk for completed suicide (Levy and Deykin, 1989). The presence of
additional risk factors only increases the level of concern and
certainty about future self-destructive acts. Thus, it is imperative that the clinician do an adequate assessment. Be-
sides inquiries about prior ideation and attempts, there
should also be a thorough exploration of drug usage patterns. What drugs are used and in what combinations, how
often are they used, and how many times has the individual
overdosed? Other risk-taking behaviors and an accident history should be obtained as well. Since the drug scene has
become increasingly violent, it is necessary to ask about access
to weapons (especially guns) and have them removed from
the patient's environment.

The presence of other psychiatric syndromes should be
followed up with adequate and appropriate treatment. In
view of the risk, it may be wise to consider brief hospitalization followed by aggressive outpatient psychotherapy, as well
as psychopharmacologic treatment of suicidal substance
abusers. The ultimate goal of treatment of the suicidal substance abuser is total abstinence from all drug use. This goal
needs to be stated and reiterated throughout treatment.

Substance abusers are notoriously difficult to treat, and
there is no simple approach. A good treatment program will
recognize the need for multiple approaches to deal with the

biomedical, psychologic, and psychosocial aspects of substance abuse. Treatment begins with detoxification and assessment of concurrent psychiatric and psychosocial problems. Other approaches include group therapy employing former users who are trained in both substance abuse and suicide counseling. Groups are a natural vehicle for providing education about the effects of substance abuse and its impact on a user's life. Individual psychotherapy can often aid in dealing with the internal tension regulation problems these patients manifest. Cognitive–behavioral approaches may be useful in helping the person develop alternative coping skills to deal with boredom, depressive states, stressful situations, and anger. Self-help groups can aid the individual in sustaining abstinence from substance abuse in the future. Family members also need education, support, and counseling about how to deal with an adolescent who is both a substance abuser and a suicide risk. They need to be told about and appreciate the heightened danger of lethality that this combination portends.

Suicide Bereavement

Until recently, suicide investigators have paid scant attention to the psychological impact on families and significant others of the self-inflicted death of a family member. From 1970 to 1985, fewer than 20 published studies of suicide family survivors were published. Recent years have seen an increased interest in this area of study, with more than 60 published papers and abstracts from 1986 to 1992. However, a comparison of this with the large number of papers on suicide indicates a continuing lack of attention to suicide survivors. Cantor (1975) suggested that the grieving process following youth suicide is qualitatively different from that seen with natural death. Barrett and Scott (1990) compared bereavement and recovery patterns in adults who had lost their spouses through suicide, accidental death, unexpected natural death, and expected natural death. Surviving spouses were interviewed after the death. There were no significant differences among groups in frequency of common bereavement reactions, including somatization, hopelessness, anger, guilt, loss of social support, and self-destructive behaviors. However, the suicide survivors suffered more feelings of being stigmatized, shamed, and abandoned. The course and quality of recovery from grief for suicide survivors in this study were not different from those for other death survivors.

The Barrett and Scott (1990) study dealt with adult spouses, and thus cannot be interpreted as applying to the parents of adolescent suicide completers. However, it is appropriate to suggest, by analogy, that parents of youth suicide victims probably also experience a bereavement process qualitatively different from that of parents who lose a child through accident or natural causes. Certainly clinical experience indicates that parents of teen suicides have great difficulty with guilt, shame, and stigmatization. They also report a sense of failure in their parenting role, and assume a degree of responsibility for the death that may be unrealistically self-punitive. This leads to behaviors such as trying to hide the true cause of the death, unrealistically clinging to the notion that the death was really an accident ("He didn't really mean to die—it must have been a mistake"), or projecting blame elsewhere (on bad companions, drugs, or the school environment). A replication of the Barrett and Scott study with the parents of adolescents who have died from suicide, accident, or natural death would offer valuable help in the treatment of youth suicide bereavement.

Relatives of suicide victims have had their lives changed unalterably and against their wills. The aftermath of suicide results in significant psychologic distress for the parents, relatives, and spouses of the deceased. Guilt, shame, stigmatization, depression, somatization, and other psychologic traumas make the effect of an unanticipated and unwelcomed death very stressful indeed. Hendin (1991b) has suggested that the trauma of suicide for the survivor is similar to post-traumatic stress disorder (PTSD). Since these survivors of suicide greatly outnumber the victims, this is a significant area for intervention and treatment.

There are several obvious issues in the treatment of teen suicide survivors. One is the provision of crisis services. Successful crisis resolution depends on early and effective crisis intervention. Unfortunately, during the crisis of a youth suicide, therapists and parents are both usually left to their own devices. This is not the time to wait for parents to ask for help. It is wise to include as many of the family members as possible in this therapeutic endeavor. Help should be offered in as proactive a fashion as possible; basic principles of crisis therapy and grief counseling should guide the therapist. The therapist should focus on the immediate problem of dealing with the loss. Helping the family define issues and short-term goals can be extremely therapeutic. It is important to be aware of the nature of the grieving process and to identify early those individual family members who appear unable to grieve. The parents may be expected to feel guilt and shame, and working through past antecedents and present manifestations is essential. The possibility of severe depression and even suicide in a surviving family member must be borne in mind. In addition, if a parent has a drug or alcohol history, the problem may be exacerbated. The short-term use of anxiolytics is helpful, as long as they are not used to avoid or postpone dealing with feelings. After the crisis situation is over, longer-term therapy may be appropriate; it can take a lifetime to get over the sequelae of a suicide.

The victim's therapist (if there was one) may have unconscious countertransference issues to deal with, as well as conscious feelings of guilt, shame, and blame (Chemtob et al., 1988). No therapist who has suffered through the suicide of a patient has escaped feelings of self-doubt and inadequacy. Many withdraw from usual social interactions; few seek or are offered brief therapy and peer consultation. A therapist who does not at least get a consultation when a patient commits suicide is leaving himself or herself open for potential problems later on.

Ron M, a third-year psychiatric resident, was treating a severely depressed borderline 18-year old woman. Dr. M was her third therapist in as many years; she had been in treatment with him for 7 stormy months. At first, therapy had gone well, with the patient considerably overidealizing her therapist. She declared that he was the first one who really understood her, and that with his guidance she would be able to make real progress. At 3 months into treatment, the patient developed an eroticized transference, which Dr. M concealed from his supervisor for several weeks. He was single, and the patient found this out. Dr. M was eventually successful in setting limits and defining the therapeutic contract, but the patient began to regress. She started drinking and using drugs again after an 8-month hiatus. She frequently showed up for therapy in an intoxicated state. When Dr. M tried to control this by insisting that it was impossible to do effective therapy when the patient was intoxicated, she missed several sessions. A letter to the patient, suggesting that she return to therapy, drop out, or accept a referral, brought her back into treatment. She was again compliant, but began to talk about her many affairs in great detail. Dr. M responded by pointing out her feelings of poor self-esteem, depression, and a pattern of self-destructive behavior. She became visibly more depressed, with biologic signs of depression. She was started on a tricyclic antidepressant and began to show improvement in her sleep pattern. At this point, Dr. M's engagement to a locally prominent woman was announced in the Sunday paper. The patient took all her remaining antidepressants and hanged herself. She was found by a friend who was worried about not seeing her for 2 days.

Dr. M's reactions to the suicide included feelings of guilt because he had not prepared the patient for the announcement of his engagement; fear of malpractice; fear that his supervisor would blame him; feelings of inadequacy; and shame because he was the only one in his group to have a patient commit suicide. Initially, he resisted meeting with his supervisor, because there was no patient to discuss. Although Dr. M was in personal therapy, the supervisor insisted that it was important educationally for him to understand what had happened and to work through his grief over the death. After several supervisory sessions, the supervisor felt that Dr. M's understanding and handling of the suicide were satisfactory, and supervision was terminated. Dr. M satisfactorily finished the residency a year later.

Parents may need a variety of kinds of support and understanding through the crisis following a child's suicide. One particularly useful intervention that has a high level of acceptability is referral to a self-help group. Self-help groups of suicide survivors provide members with mutual assistance in working through the trauma of suicide and continuing on with their lives. Such groups offer a point of connection, help members overcome feelings of helplessness, and, through the understanding they provide of a shared experience, can be a source of ego reinforcement. The local suicide prevention service or the national self-help clearinghouse may be able to provide the therapist with the details on locally available suicide survivor groups. The American Association of Suicidology has a catalog of resources for survivors of suicide; books, videotapes, and a newsletter are listed. A directory of suicide survivor support groups in the United States and Canada is also available from this same source (American Association of Suicidology, 2459 South Ash Street, Denver, Colorado 80222).

OTHER INTERVENTIONS AND PREVENTION

The purpose of this section is to explore other intervention strategies and prevention strategies for youth suicide. Several reviews deal with various aspects of intervention and prevention of suicide among youth; the work of five groups of reviewers is discussed here (Blumenthal and Kupfer, 1988; Rosenberg et al., 1987, 1989; *Report of the Secretary's Task Force on Youth Suicide*, 1989; Shaffer et al., 1988; Holinger and Offer, 1986, and Holinger, 1990a). These reviews demonstrate a wide range of approaches, from new conceptions of early detection (Blumenthal and Kupfer, 1988) to descriptions of interventions with estimates of potential lives saved (Rosenberg et al., 1987, 1989) to specific prevention and postvention strategies (Shaffer et al., 1988).

Levels of Detection:
Blumenthal and Kupfer's Work

Blumenthal and Kupfer (1988) described five overlapping domains of risk factors for suicide among youth: family history and genetics; personality traits; psychosocial life events and chronic medical illness; psychiatric disorder; and biologic factors. The authors then described three different levels of detection. Level 1, termed "detection awareness," refers to detection of individuals who are not actively suicidal or in immediate danger of suicide completion but who do have certain risk factors. These include being (a) the offspring of affectively ill or substance-abusing parents; (b) the offspring of suicides and suicide attempters; (c) the close contacts of suicides and suicidal people; (d) abused and neglected children; and (e) children who have recently been under severe stress. Level 2, termed "major problem awareness," refers to detection of major problems (e.g., academic problems, self-esteem and sexual identity problems, running away, an unwanted pregnancy, etc.) that do not meet DSM-III-R criteria for a psychiatric disorder; however, young individuals who fit into Level 2 may require assessment, intervention, and perhaps even treatment. Level 3, termed "major psychiatric disorder," refers (as the name implies) to the detection of suicidal youth who have major psychiatric disorders. The two elements of Level 3 include (a) appropriate assessment and evaluation, and (b) a treatment component aimed at the specific psychiatric diagnosis (e.g., affective disorder, schizophrenia, substance abuse, etc.).

Estimates of Possible Benefit: Rosenberg et al.'s Work

Rosenberg et al. (1987) described several intervention and prevention strategies and attempted to estimate the numbers of lives that could be saved with each. For example, they suggested that limiting the availability of lethal agents could markedly reduce the suicide rates. They estimated that if access to handguns were reduced for the general population, some 5,370 suicides a year would be prevented. If access to firearms were limited only for persons with major psychiatric disorders, approximately 1,100 suicides would be prevented. If legislation restricting the amount of medication given at any one time were passed, approximately 750 lives would be saved each year. Additional training of "gatekeepers" (e.g., clergy, primary care physicians, teachers, etc.) with respect to suicide and other self-destructive behaviors was estimated to result in a saving of about 750 lives per year. Finally, better responsiveness to demographic variables and suicide epidemics could result in preventing 825 suicides per year.

Rosenberg et al. (1989) also contacted researchers and clinicians in the field of youth suicide and asked them what preventive interventions would be most effective. Restricting access to firearms and identifying high-risk youth were deemed to be the two most potentially effective interventions. These were followed, in order of endorsement, by improved treatment, school-based screening, crisis centers and hotlines, effective education, restricting access to medications, and restricting access to high places.

Recommendations of the Secretary's Task Force on Youth Suicide

The U.S. Department of Health and Human Services' Secretary's Task Force on Youth Suicide carried out an exhaustive 2-year study of risk factors and intervention strategies in youth suicide, and its final recommendations (*Report of the Secretary's Task Force on Youth Suicide*, 1989) are well worth noting. The task force made six major recommendations, the first two dealing with enhancing the understanding of the problem and the last four with intervention and prevention strategies. Recommendation 1 was to develop accurate, timely, and valid data on suicide and attempted suicide, including (a) uniform criteria for suicide; (b) data on community-based surveillance systems for suicide attempts; and (c) data on unusual suicide patterns (e.g., clusters). Recommendation 2 was to conduct multidisciplinary research to determine and evaluate the risk factors for suicide, including (a) risk factors suggested by surveillance data and biobehavioral factors; (b) antecedent risk factors; and (c) suicide clusters and contagion. Recommendation 3 was to evaluate the effectiveness and cost of interventions to prevent suicide. These included interventions addressed to the general population, ones addressed to specific populations, and ones intended to limit access of youth to lethal means of suicide. Recommendation 4 was to support the delivery of suicide prevention services, especially by increasing the numbers and training of professionals and paraprofessionals in work with suicidal young people. Recommendation 5 was to inform and educate the public and health service providers about current knowledge in the prevention, diagnosis, and treatment of suicide among youth. Finally, Recommendation 6, termed "Broader Approaches," suggested involving both public and private sectors in the prevention of youth suicide. This included a variety of strategies to involve business, philanthropy, the criminal and juvenile justice systems, and other organizations and agencies in the task of preventing youth suicide.

Specific Prevention/Postvention Strategies: Shaffer et al.'s Work

The discussion of prevention of youth suicide by Shaffer's group (1988) was preceded by a description of a model for suicide causation. According to these authors, the two key issues of individual predisposition (e.g., psychopathology) and social milieu combine with "trigger factors" to precipitate a suicide. These "trigger factors" include stress events, altered states of mind (e.g., intoxication or rage), and opportunity (e.g., access to a method).

Shaffer et al. divided their intervention strategies into primary, secondary, and tertiary prevention, with postvention as a separate category. Under primary prevention, they highlighted providing psychiatric services and restricting methods used to commit suicide; they also discussed in detail the controversial issue of the effectiveness of school-based programs. Their secondary and tertiary interventions included providing hotline and crisis services and treating suicide attempters. Under postvention strategies they described various possible interventions following a suicide, such as treatment for the survivors (family, friends, etc.) and preventing contagion at the school.

Different Strategies, Different Groups: Our Own Work

We have also reviewed intervention and prevention strategies for suicidal youth (Holinger and Offer, 1986; Holinger, 1990a). We addressed two major target goups (the general population and high-risk populations) and three types of strategies (primary, secondary, and tertiary prevention strategies).

The first area within primary prevention was termed "developmental aspects." As we have noted earlier in this chapter, current infant research and the study of affects have productively challenged older theories and helped clarify much about what human beings feel, why they feel it, and how they communicate it. Our recommendations included studies on the impact of the following: school classes dealing with this topic; the training of teachers; and parents obtaining this information via the schools, obstetricians, and other physicians. The second area of primary prevention involves the suicide assessment training of various professional groups—not only psychiatrists, but other physicians (internists, family practitioners, obstetricians, etc.), social workers, clergy, and so forth. The third area involves the restriction of lethal agents. Guns and medications are currently among the most common causes of successful overt suicide (as noted throughout the present book), and we reviewed the controversy surrounding possible regulation of these agents in both the general population and high-risk groups. The fourth area involves suicide prevention centers. Although the success of such organizations and centers is controversial, Miller et al. (1984) found that such centers consistently reduced the suicide rates of young white females by approximately 1.75 deaths per 100,000 population. The fifth area involves studies of population changes and cohort effects. This area includes the implications of demographic variables for the prediction, intervention, and prevention of suicide and is described more fully in Chapter 9.

Secondary prevention, as we reviewed it, refers to intervention and involves suicide attempters (discussed in more detail in connection with the high-risk populations).

Tertiary prevention, or postprevention, refers to efforts directed toward those people and institutions (e.g., schools) who have been psychologically close to adolescents who committed suicide. Clinically, tertiary prevention involves family members and friends; on an epidemiologic level, such prevention takes the form of preventing epidemics of suicide.

We also discussed two high-risk populations. The first high-risk population includes psychiatric patients and suicide attempters, and various preventive and intervention strategies for such individuals were described. The second high-risk group is defined by sociodemographic variables (e.g., being single, divorced, or widowed; being unemployed; and coming from a younger age group in the "baby boom" generation).

Since these reports were published, additional studies have been conducted on the potential of gun control to decrease both suicide and homicide rates. For example, Brent et al. (1991) found that the presence of a gun in the house was a statistically significant risk factor for youth suicide, regardless of how effectively that gun was stored. Previously, Kellerman and Reay (1986) had studied 398 cases of deaths by guns kept in the homes for self-protection; only 2% of the deaths were caused by the guns' being fired for self-protection, whereas in 84% the guns were used for suicide. On a larger level, a comparison of Seattle and Vancouver suggested that stricter Canadian gun control laws were associated with significantly lower suicide and homicide rates for young people (Cotton, 1992). Loftin et al. (1991) obtained similar results for both suicide and homicide among adults in Washington, D.C., following the institution in 1976 of a very restrictive gun control law. The relationship between gun control and youthful suicide and homicide is critical (e.g., see Kassirer, 1991; Zimring, 1991) and involves large numbers of people: Not only are a consistently high proportion of youth suicide and homicide victims killed by guns, but a recent Centers for Disease Control (CDC) study showed that in any given month approximately 525,000 U.S. high school students occasionally carry a gun (CDC, 1991).

SUMMARY

Treatment of the suicidal adolescent is still largely an empirical art. There are few controlled studies of efficacy, particularly scientifically controlled ones, to guide the clinician. The vast range of behaviors and diagnoses, and the frequency of comorbidity, increase the challenge. Moreover, families are not always willing collaborators in treatment. Thus, the clinician is advised to assume a pragmatic posture and remain flexible. The specific treatment approach to the adolescent suicide attempter will depend upon the clinician's (or, in the case of an inpatient setting, the milieu's) experience and treatment philosophy. Regardless of whether a clinician is doing family, group, or individual therapy, it may be useful to develop a treatment plan with defined goals; the plan should be kept flexible and updated as treatment progresses. In addition, it is important to know how to survive the suicide of a patient and how to help the family survivors of suicide grieve and then carry on with their lives.

The present discussion of the assessment and treatment of suicidal youth also seems to show the overlap and importance of both the clinical and epidemiologic perspectives. Such epidemiologic risk factors as presence of a major psychiatric disorder, substance abuse, sexual identity problems, behavioral problems, gun availability, and so on are critical in assessing suicidality. It would appear that a combined use of epidemiologic and clinical data would best serve the clinician in the very difficult task of treating suicidal youth.

Finally, a study of several reviews of interventions and prevention of youth suicide reveals many different approaches. However, four strategies tend to be consistently viewed as potentially effective: some form of firearms control, public education, training of professionals, and research.

CHAPTER EIGHT

Homicide: Intervention and Prevention

Most data for youth homicide are still sociocultural; unlike the situation with youth suicide, little evidence exists regarding the psychologic character structure of victims or perpetrators. Victims and perpetrators share similar characteristics. Youth homicide is especially frequent among nonwhites, especially African-Americans. Contrary to popular opinion, domestic violence is still the most frequent cause of youth homicide: Victim and perpetrator usually know each other. Poverty appears to be the most consistent underlying risk factor in communities with high homicide rates. Less research is available for homicide prevention than for suicide prevention. Various forms of primary, secondary, and tertiary prevention strategies are explored, with an emphasis on intervening at various levels of the cycle of domestic violence.

A study of some of the clinical issues of youth homicide again demonstrates the importance of the epidemiologic–clinical interaction. On the macroscopic level, epidemiologic findings such as research data and generalizations gleaned from specific cases are critical to informing policy and research decisions for clinical medicine, services, and so on. On a microscopic level, the understanding of the circumstances of homicide will seriously influence how both potential victims and potential and actual perpetrators can best be assessed and treated in efforts to prevent and intervene in homicide situations. In this chapter, following a brief background section, various etiologic issues are raised, including types of homicide, poverty, and biologic factors. Intervention and prevention strategies and programs are then discussed, and many of these provide further insights into the problem of youth homicide. Both victims and perpetrators of youth homicide are discussed, and it should be noted at the outset that their characteristics are quite similar.

BACKGROUND

As noted in previous chapters, the overall suicide and homicide rates among youth have been rather similar over the years, although the past few years have seen somewhat higher homicide rates. For 15- to 19-year-olds in 1990, the total suicide rate is 11.1 per 100,000, and the homicide rate is 17.0; for 20- to 24-year-olds, the suicide rate is 15.1, and the homicide rate is 22.5. In addition, the shifts in rates over time for youth suicide and homicide are similar (see Chapter 4). However, when we look more closely at the epidemiologic and clinical data, differences emerge that have profound implications for treatment and preventive strategies.

One of the most striking differences is the racial/ethnic distribution of adolescent homicide victims and perpetrators. Whereas the suicide rates for white youth are approximately twice those for nonwhites, the homicide pattern is the reverse, and the differences are far greater. The 1990 homicide rate for nonwhite males 15–24 years of age is 109.1 per 100,000—more than seven times the rate for white males (15.4 per 100,000); for nonwhite and white females in that same age range, the difference is nearly fourfold (15.5 per 100,000 and 4.0 per 100,000, respectively) (see Chapter 4). As Christoffel (1990) has noted, although more than half of all homicide victims are white, African-American homicide rates far exceed those for whites at all ages. African-American male rates compared to white male rates are four times higher in infancy, three times higher in the 1- to 4-year-old, 5- to 9-year-old, and 10- to 14-year-old groups, and more than six times higher in the 15- to 19-year-old age group. Furthermore, Christoffel has observed that homicide was the only leading cause of childhood death in the United States that increased during the post-World War II decades.

The evidence suggests that inner-city Latino youth have homicide rates comparable to those of African-Americans. For example, in Chicago the yearly murder rate between 1987 and 1989 for Latino males between the ages of 14 and 29 was 102 per 100,000, compared to 152 per 100,000 for African-Americans and 17 per 100,000 for whites. However, among 15- to 19-year-olds the African-American and Latino murder rates were identical: 126 per 100,000 (Block, 1993).

More than in any other age group, adolescent homicides are likely to be committed with a firearm (Christoffel, 1990). In 1988, the firearm death rate for African-American males 15–19 years old was 2.6 times that from natural causes. In that same year, firearm death rates for white males in this age group exceeded those from natural causes for the first time (Fingerhut et al., 1991). Racial comparisons indicate that African-American youth are much more likely than white youth to die by means of a firearm: In 1988, African-American males aged 15–19 had a firearm homicide rate 11 times that of white males. However, paralleling racial differences in suicide, the firearm suicide rate for white males was twice that for African-American males (12.7 and 6.8, respectively) in that same year and same age range (Fingerhut et al., 1991).

Predictably, an examination of perpetration of homicide shows ethnic and racial patterns similar to those of victimization. For example, youth under 18 account for slightly more than 10% of all homicide perpetrators, but African-Americans account for 50% and Latinos account for 25% of those arrested (whereas African-Americans and Latinos represent only about 15% and 4% of the juvenile population, respectively). When we examine youth who perpetrate homicide, it is important to remember that youth often kill in groups, and, as a result, will account for a greater percentage of homicide arrests than of homicide victimization rates.

Certain states have higher homicide rates than others, and these rates also vary by race and ethnicity. In 1987, the states with the highest white male homicide rates per 100,000 for the 15–24 age range were California (22.0), Texas (20.9), New York (18.4), Arizona (17.4), and Florida (15.4). Among states with large African-American populations, those with the highest African-American homicide rates per 100,000 were Michigan (231.6), California (155.3), New York (136.5), and Missouri (130.5). Thus, Michigan, with the highest young African-American male homicide rate, has a rate 10 times that of California, with the highest young white male homicide rate (Fingerhut and Kleinman, 1990).

Clearly, homicide for nonwhite youth ranks higher than any other cause of death for any youthful ethnic and racial group (Krause et al., 1988). For this reason, the following section tends to focus on the homicide issues involving nonwhite youth. In addition, in youth homicide research there is a paucity of detailed psychologic autopsy studies, which have contributed so importantly to our understanding of youth suicide. This problem exists for both victims and perpetrators of homicide. Thus, the next section provides a broader social perspective. Treatment implications are discussed more fully in the section on intervention and prevention.

ETIOLOGIC CONSIDERATIONS

A majority of adolescent homicide victims and perpetrators have similar characteristics (McDermott, 1983; Jensen and Bronsonfield, 1986; Uehara et al., in press). The victims and perpetrators of homicide tend to be about the same age, to be members of the same ethnic group, and to know each other as peers or acquaintances. Furthermore, both groups may have histories of previous victimizations or histories of witnessing violence. The circumstances of many adolescent homicides—that is, interpersonal altercations ("expressive homicides"; see below)—suggest that many youthful victims and perpetrators live in a violent milieu in which the role of victim or perpetrator depends on the chance outcome of the altercation. Victims and perpetrators both show a propensity to engage in physical altercations more commonly than usual. Thus, it becomes necessary to study both victims' and perpetrators' characteristics in order to get a full understanding of the problem of youth homicide. Analogous findings have been obtained regarding the characteristics of adult homicide victims and perpetrators (Dennis et al., 1981; Rose, 1981), in that both groups show a propensity for getting into physical altercations more commonly than usual, and their characteristics are more similar than dissimilar. Table 8.1 summarizes the characteristics of both victims and perpetrators of youth homicide.

Types of Homicide

According to Christoffel (1990), youth homicide victimization falls into two basic categories: "infantile" and "adolescent." The infantile pattern occurs with children under age 5; the perpetrator is most often a parent or caretaker, and the circumstances involve discipline of a child, which escalates to child abuse and then to homicide. The adolescent pattern occurs with children and youth over age 11; the perpetrators are most often peers, acquaintances, or possibly

TABLE 8.1. Youth Homicide: Characteristics of Both Victims and Perpetrators

---

Rates
   Nonwhites have much higher rates than whites
   Males have much higher rates than females
   Teens have more "gang-related" homicides than adults

Etiologic associations
   Poverty
   Acquired biologic factors
   Gun availability
   Various character pathologies?

Type of homicide and ethnicity
   African-American: Expressive > gang > instrumental
   Hispanic: Gang > instrumental > expressive
   White: Gang > expressive > instrumental

---

gangs (most commonly among Latinos), and the circumstances involve an interpersonal altercation. Latency-age children may be a victim of either pattern. The most common lethal means in infantile murders are beatings, whereas for adolescent murders the most common lethal means is gunshot.

Another useful means of classifying homicides focuses more on the motivation of the perpetration. "Expressive homicides," which account for the majority of all homicides, are defined as crimes of rage or passion that usually occur between family members, friends, or acquaintances. "Instrumental homicides" are committed during a felony such as robbery, and usually involve strangers (Block, 1993). A category that is particularly useful in regard to youth is that of "gang-related homicide," which has elements of both instrumental and expressive homicide but is motivated by gang activity or gang membership (Block, 1993). The distinctions among these types of homicide syndromes are important in understanding homicide rates in various groups, as well as in developing intervention and prevention strategies.

An illustration of the ethnic and age variations in these syndromes is provided by analyses of homicide data from Chicago from 1982 to 1989 (Block, 1993; Jenkins and Bell, 1992). Among 15- to 19-year-old males, gang-related deaths accounted for 65% of the homicides for Hispanic youth, compared to 48% for white youth and 34% for African-American youth. On the other hand, expressive violence accounted for 41% of the homicides of African-American youth, compared to 27% for white youth and only 15% for Latino youth (Jenkins and Bell, 1992). Offender profiles are similar, with the interesting exception that although African-American youth are more likely to be gang violence victims than victims of instrumental violence, they are somewhat more likely to be perpetrators of instrumental violence than gang violence, and are most likely to perpetrate expressive violence (Block, 1993).

In general, the circumstances of youth perpetration of homicide are similar to the circumstances for adults. In reviewing juvenile homicides during 1984, Ewing (1990) noted that victims of juvenile homicide were similar to victims of adult homicide. Parents/stepparents accounted for 8.3%, other family members for 9.4%, acquaintances for 49%, and strangers for 33% of the victims (with 58% of the victims who were strangers being victims of a felony crime [instrumental violence] prior to the homicide). Both Ewing (1990) and Benedek and Cornell (1989) found that children who killed a parent either had been abused by that parent or had a history of extended interpersonal conflict with the victim.

Regarding the mental states of youthful homicide perpetrators, most researchers agree that few are psychotic or mentally retarded, although many have learning difficulties (Busch et al., 1990). Some experts in the area, most notably Lewis et al. (1985), maintain that these children are more likely to have symptoms of neurologic difficulties and transient, nonschizophrenic psychotic symptoms. Although there are risk factors that are more prevalent in homicide offenders, there are no known personality types associated with homicide in adults or children; again, the majority of these homicides begin with interpersonal altercations, and such episodes are likely to occur over the total range of personality types.

Poverty

Various theorists have attempted to explain the disproportionately high rate of homicide among African-Americans, which since the beginning of the 20th century has been 5 to 10 times higher than that for any other group (Holinger, 1987). One hypothesis, entitled the "subculture-of-violence theory," proposes that certain African-Americans have a subculture (developed from the violence of slavery; racism; and the effects of discrimination, unemployment, and poverty) that not only tolerates violence but expects and promotes it (Wolfgang and Ferracuti, 1967). This theory arose from the finding that the inner-city environment produces a type of murderer who is characteristically young,

African-American, poor, and quick to respond aggressively to narcissistic injury. However, the usefulness of this theory is questionable. The violent behavior that has become distressingly frequent in many inner-city neighborhoods could simply be attributed to behavioral adaptations of some individuals, and not to a value system that permeates African-American culture (Willie, 1985).

A more reasonable explanation seems to be that the disproportionately high rate of homicide among African-Americans is not based on subcultural, racial, or ethnic factors, but on situational sociologic factors that relate to poverty. Research has shown that poverty is an underlying risk factor for death by homicide (Flango and Sherbonou, 1976; Williams, 1984; Loftin and Hill, 1974), and that when socioeconomic status is held constant, the racial differences in homicide rates decrease substantially (University of California at Los Angeles and Centers For Disease Control, 1985; Tardiff, 1987). One reason why controlling for poverty does not completely equalize homicide rates between African-Americans and whites may be that poor African-Americans and whites live in different contexts. Poor African-Americans tend to be concentrated in ghettos, whereas poor whites tend to be in more diverse neighborhoods. Thus, the variables associated with poverty and likely to increase homicide tend to be more concentrated where poor African-Americans, rather than poor whites live. Another observation that supports the importance of the poverty factor is the finding that the homicide rate among civilian African-American male populations is 12 times higher than the rate of African-American males in the Army (Rothberg et al., 1990). Certainly a subcultural variable would not stop exerting its influence simply because the sociologic environment changed.

Furthermore, it is suggested that the contribution of poverty to African-American adolescent violence is one of relative rather than absolute deprivation (Hawkins, 1986; Freiburg, 1991). African-American and Latino youth, 40%-45% of whom live in poverty-level families (U.S. Bureau of the Census, 1990), have the highest unemployment rates in the country. In our consumer-oriented society, where individual worth is often defined by personal acquisitions, the mass media create tastes; in areas where extreme poverty and wealth exist in close proximity, poor youth may be particularly frustrated by "not having," and hence may be vulnerable to involvement in lucrative but dangerous activities. In addition, the adolescent tendency toward risk taking is often more extreme in poor youth, who may use such behaviors to compensate for barriers to achievement in the more traditional areas of academic, career, athletic, and/or family success.

Many other factors cited to explain the relatively high murder rates among African-American youth are also related to poverty. These include the increase in children born to inexperienced teen mothers, many of whom lack adequate parenting skills and physical resources, and an increase in drug use. The latter contributes to neglect and abuse of youngsters, as well as to an increase in instrumental and gang-related violence among youth. Also, it has been noted that the number of minority youth is increasing—a demographic factor that, even in the absence of an increase in other risk factors, may contribute to an increase in the number of youth homicides (Holinger, 1987).

Biologic Factors

Biologic factors may be among the more underrated contributors to the high rates of African-American youth homicide. Head injury and consequent central nervous system damage may increase violence by increasing limbic-mediated violence and/or decreasing cerebral restraint of violence (Bell, 1986, 1987). Neurologic damage also contributes to learning disabilities, which, as noted, may be related to aggressive behavior. The effects may be compounded by sociologic variables, such as poor housing, poor nutrition, and poor health care. Research has shown that head injury (e.g., resulting from falls, recreational accidents, and automobile accidents) is more prevalent among male children (with peaks in midadolescence), the poor, and African-Americans (Rivara and Mueller, 1986). Consequently, poor African-American male children are at greatest risk for head injury and its consequences.

In summary, although far too little is known about youth homicide, the above-described studies do suggest many treatment options—that is, intervention and prevention strategies. The outcomes of such strategies as they have been implemented to date also teach much about youth homicide, and various intervention and prevention issues are discussed in detail below.

INTERVENTION/PREVENTION PROGRAMS AND STRATEGIES

The purpose of this section is to study the extensive programs and strategies in place in U.S. communities that are intended to reduce the rate of youth homicide. Interestingly, much information about youth homicide emerges from this work, as many of these studies are, in effect, "natural experiments" (MacMahon and Pugh, 1970).

Prior to the implementation of specific strategies for the prevention of homicide, considerable education is needed to raise the consciousness of various segments of society regarding the issue. As an example, let us take the problem of homicide among young African-Americans, inasmuch as their rates are so high. Such awareness and education must focus on destroying certain myths about African-American homicide while creating an understanding of its actual dynamics, developing African-American community ownership of the problem, stimulating self-help initiatives, and developing a commitment for policy and action. Primary target groups are the African-American community, which is eventually responsible for implementing strategies, and policy makers, who can stimulate activity in an area mainly through their appropriation of funds and technical assistance (Bell and Jenkins, 1990). The initial goal of an education and awareness campaign must be to increase the African-American community's understanding and ownership of the problem. First of all, some African-Americans are simply not aware of the extent of the problem. Although most African-American people "feel" that African-Americans are more likely than whites to die violently, they may be genuinely shocked at the magnitude of the difference. These numbers need to be publicized in a meaningful and impactful manner—that is, in comparison to the numbers for whites, as well as in relationship to the numbers of African-Americans who die from other causes, such as AIDS and sickle cell anemia. Community-based organizations and conferences (e.g., the Black-on-Black Love Campaign in Chicago, Save Our Sons and Daughters in Detroit, Blacks Mobilized Against Crime in Richmond, Virginia, and the Association of Black Social Workers Anti-Violence Program in New Orleans) have started the process of educating the public. African-American-oriented radio stations are ideally situated to help raise consciousness in regard to this issue. Writings on young victims and on the exposure of inner-city children to violence bring a human face to the statistics and allow individuals to connect emotionally to the issue (e.g., Kotlowitz, 1987, 1991).

The planning of violence prevention and intervention strategies must also take into account of the type of violence that is most prevalent in the group of interest. As noted previously, a useful classification system is the one focusing on the motivation of the perpetrator (expressive, instrumental, or gang-related). The prevalence of these types of violence vary by age group, ethnicity, and locale, as well as across time. Thus, a necessary first step in designing an intervention strategy is to establish a surveillance system that monitors the characteristics and circumstances of violence within a community. In general, for African-American youth most homicides are expressive in nature, although gang-related and instrumental homicides are increasing dramatically; for Latino youth, the predominant type of homicide is gang-related.

Just as the types of violence can be classified, so can the intervention strategies. Steps taken to prevent a problem from occurring are referred to as forms of "primary prevention." "Secondary prevention" and "tertiary prevention," in contrast, take place after the onset of the "illness" in the early and late stages, respectively. Obviously, the most effective homicide prevention strategies are those that occur before the incident; however, as discussed below, secondary strategies applied when violent behavior situations have already occurred can still prevent the occurrence of more extreme and lethal violence. The various prevention strategies are summarized in Table 8.2.

Primary Prevention

Primary prevention strategies are tied to the causes of homicide and include a number of approaches, including

TABLE 8.2. Prevention/Intervention Strategies in Youth Homicide

Primary prevention
  Decreases in poverty (improved economic conditions for the poor, creation of jobs, etc.)
  Public education about the youth homicide problem (its causes, prevention, and interventions)
  Improvement of conflict resolution skills
  Creation of community and school enrichment programs
  Improvement and stabilization of family systems
  Reduction of acquired biologic factors that enhance impulsivity (alcohol, head injury, etc.)
  Firearms control
  Strengthening of ethnic identity

Secondary prevention
  Identification and treatment of potential victims and perpetrators of sublethal violence who may be at risk for being homicide victims or perpetrators
  Effective intervention in violent situations
    Training police, doctors, counselors, clergy, etc., in how to assist in violence intervention
    Providing emergency room services for domestic disputes and other forms of expressive violence

Tertiary prevention
  Treatment of those exposed to homicide, as covictims and/or witnesses
  Treatment of perpetrators

improvement of conflict resolution skills, creation of community and school enrichment programs, improvement and stabilization of family systems, reduction in acquired biologic contributors to violence, control of firearms, and strengthening of racial identity. It is interesting to note that the Centers for Disease Control have recently issued a publication describing many such programs aimed at preventing youth violence (National Center for Injury Prevention and Control, 1993). The increasing importance and public acceptance of these programs seem demonstrated by such a publication.

Improvement of Conflict Resolution Skills

As noted previously, most homicides occur as a result of altercations among acquaintances, fueled by emotion and anger. Violence erupts as individuals get locked into an escalating situation from which it is difficult to extricate themselves without loss of face, and which they lack skills other than violence for defusing. Some individuals apparently have a propensity for this; again as noted earlier, homicide victims and perpetrators have a higher frequency of involvement in physical altercations than do others (Dennis et al., 1981; Rose, 1981). For these individuals, the development of skills to handle interpersonal conflict in a nonviolent, constructive manner should be especially useful for reducing their involvement in violent and potentially violent encounters.

Several programs that reduce violence through knowledge and skill building are currently in place and have had some apparent success (Wilson-Brewer et al., 1990; Prothrow-Stith, 1986). For example the Violence Prevention Curriculum for Adolescents, in place in Boston high schools, teaches adolescents to deal constructively with anger and potentially violent situations. The school program consists of a ten-session course presented to high school students in a structured curriculum format. Operating from the perspective that most violence is expressive (i.e., the result of an angry outburst), and that individuals make choices about their behavior, the curriculum addresses three broad issues: the role of anger in violence (including the recognition that anger is legitimate) and ways of addressing anger without violence; risk factors associated with violence and youth homicide; and nonviolent conflict resolution techniques (Prothrow-Stith, 1986; Wilson-Brewer et al., 1990).

A similar program that uses African-American actors and culturally relevant situations has been developed for use with African-American youth (Hammond and Yung, 1991). Entitled *Anger: Working It Out,* the videotape program discusses three conflict resolution skills: "Givin' it," "Takin' it," and "Workin' it out." The "Givin' it" skill focuses on calmly and clearly explaining one's grievance to the offending party; the "Takin' it" skill teaches how to take criticism calmly from another party; and the "Workin' it out" skill focuses on negotiation.

Most such programs are grounded in a cognitive or information-processing approach to aggression, which focuses on the system of beliefs and the cognitive processing skills that support and maintain aggressive behavior. One such model (Dodge, 1986; Slaby and Guerra, 1988) proposes that childhood and adolescent aggression can result from biases in information processing at any of five steps: (1) selective attention to cues and the amount of information that is sought about a situation (aggressive youth seek less information about a situation); (2) defining the problem and selecting goals (aggressive and possibly victimized youth are more likely to define situations as hostile, and to choose strategies of defense accordingly); (3) response search, or generating solutions to the problem (aggressive youth generate fewer solutions); (4) response decision, where the individual considers the consequences of his or her actions; and (5) enactment. In addition, it has been found that aggressive youth have a system of aggression-supporting beliefs, including the belief that aggression is legitimate and that it enhances self-esteem and status among their peers (Slaby and Guerra, 1988; Guerra and Slaby, 1990).

An explicit test of this cognitive processing approach is the Viewpoints Training Program, currently based at the

University of Illinois–Chicago Center for Research on Aggression (Guerra and Slaby, 1990). The program, tested at a California state juvenile correctional center on youth who had committed one or more violent crimes, is designed to alter in 12 weekly 1-hour sessions the previously mentioned beliefs that support violence and the information processing that precedes the decision to act violently. Participants are taught to evaluate the situation ("Is there a problem?"), gather information, generate nonviolent solutions, and evaluate the consequences of their actions. Beliefs are changed by having participants write arguments refuting their original beliefs and presenting them to the group. Evaluation of the program found that the participants, in comparison to a control group from the same institution, showed improved problem-solving skills, less aggressive beliefs, and less aggression as reported by the staff at the facility. Recidivism figures at 12- and 24-month follow-ups found that program participants were less likely, but not significantly so, to violate their parole. This latter finding highlights the difficulty in translating attitude change into behavioral change, and, probably most importantly, the difficulty in maintaining the new behaviors and attitudes in the old setting.

The placement of violence prevention curricula in primary and secondary schools is critical. School-based programs, particularly in early grades, insure that all students are exposed to the information (many of the most troubled students may have left the system by high school). In addition, a classroom approach can establish norms for the group, which members then use as a standard for evaluating one another's behavior. Ideally, norms of competitiveness and face saving through aggression can be replaced with a norm of nonviolence that is reinforced by the group. Group members no longer expect and urge one another to fight, as this has ceased to be the appropriate behavior.

Although structured institutionalized programs are becoming increasingly popular, it should be noted that less structured approaches can also be effective. For example, the use of humor (if it is not at one's adversary's expense) can often defuse a potentially violent situation. Pretending not to hear the person and asking him or her to repeat the insult can be quite effective, as the repeated insult will be less venomous. With a little assistance, students can generate additional such techniques (which have the added benefit of increased credibility with the youngsters and possibly greater applicability to their specific situations). The goal of all of these techniques is to move students to an awareness and appreciation of "win–win" situations, in which outcomes acceptable to both parties can often be reached.

Creation of Community and School Enrichment Programs

Community- or school-based enrichment programs that provide a sense of direction for youth can be quite successful in altering attitudes and lifestyles that predispose them to involvement in gangs, drugs, and violence. For example, Sister Fattah's House of Umoja in Philadelphia offers vocational training, in an atmosphere of "faith and love," that provides young males with a legitimate means of making money to replace their involvement in less legitimate and more dangerous enterprises. Similar programs exist throughout the country (Sulton, 1987; Wilson-Brewer et al., 1990); they are typically aimed at reducing youth's involvement in gangs, drugs, and violence by enhancing their self-esteem, improving their conflict resolution skills, and encouraging and/or providing education and job training in a supportive yet disciplined environment.

Comer (1980) of Yale has spent considerable time developing a form of "intervention research"—an intervention that actively involves various elements in a community in working together to provide a high-quality education for their children—and has looked at the outcome. His results regarding improvement in the New Haven, Connecticut, school system's educational accomplishments for poor African-American children at risk have been well documented (Comer, 1988a). Although the hypothesis that similar interventions reduce school violence has never been tested, we suspect that this type of intervention, (i.e., community–school linkages) will lower the rates of occurrence of school violence, as it seems to have done in the New Haven schools (Comer, 1988b).

Improvement and Stabilization of Family Systems

Some families under stress, particularly if they are isolated and without support, experience considerable intrafamilial violence (Gelles, 1987). Such stress may manifest itself as child abuse (the murder of young children, which is the second leading cause of death for African-American children aged 1 to 4, typically starts as physical abuse), elder abuse, and/or other types of domestic violence. Social supports that reduce the isolation and tension of these families greatly diminish the potential for abuse and violence. Drop-in day care programs for children and the elderly, as well as respite care programs for the elderly, reduce some of the stress resulting from intense involvement with a dependent family member. Home visitation programs in which nurses and paraprofessionals provide parental training and support to high-risk mothers have been effective in reducing child abuse and neglect in these families (Olds and Kitzman, 1990), and have the potential for directly decreasing the socialization of aggressive behavior by teaching parents non-violent discipline techniques.

Parenting classes, particularly for young, single mothers (who are often the most emotionally burdened), can also prevent both the injury of children and the socialization of aggressive children. As we have noted in earlier chapters, tremendous advances have been made in understanding infant development over the past decade (e.g., Stern, Lichtenberg, Emde, Brazelton, and others), and this information needs to be conveyed to parents. Such classes can also provide specific information on how to produce less aggressive children, such as the simple act of rocking an infant, which stimulates brain development and improves impulse control

(Prescott, 1975). Whatever "nurturing" services are available for families—parenting classes, respite care, family counseling, and home visitation programs—must be publicized to the community, with the understanding that families most in need, because of their isolation and stress, may be the most difficult to reach.

Reduction in Acquired Biologic Contributors to Violence

As indicated previously, head injury and subsequent neurologic damage are implicated in aggressive behavior, particularly explosive violence (Bell, 1986, 1987). The treatments for aggression that stems in part from traumatic brain injury include psychopharmacologic, behavioral, and psychologic treatments, along with social interventions (Silver et al., 1987; Corrigan et al., 1993). Medications that are felt to temper aggression secondary to head injury are carbamazepine, beta-adrenergic blocking agents, and possibly lithium. Behavior modification techniques and improved resolution of psychologic issues are useful for these patients.

Control of Firearms

As noted earlier, more homicides in adolescence than in any other age group are committed with a handgun (Christoffel, 1990; Fingerhut et al., 1991). Although firearm fatalities have increased dramatically since 1960, the greatest increase has been among youth (Christoffel, 1991). Therefore, any discussion of reducing adolescent murder must address the issue of youth access to guns (Cotton, 1992; *Journal of the American Medical Association,* 1992).

Although studies that attempt to measure the severity of the problem of kids carrying guns may be methodologically weak, because they are based on self-reports, these studies suggest reason for serious concern. For example, in a survey of 1,035 students from four high schools and two middle

schools in Chicago, 33% of the students reported that they
had carried a weapon. Of these, 63% had carried a knife,
17% a gun, and 20% some other weapon. Furthermore, 12%
indicated they had injured someone with a knife or gun
(Uehara et al., in press). In Baltimore, half of the high school
males reported that they had carried a handgun to school
(Runyan and Gerken, 1989). The National Adolescent Student Health Survey (American School Health Association,
1988) found that 41% of the boys and 24% of the girls
surveyed claimed to have easy access to a handgun. The
National School Safety Center (personal communication,
1991) estimates that on any given day 90,000 boys are carrying a gun. As suggested by these surveys, most youth who
carry guns to school do not carry semiautomatic or automatic
weapons, contrary to popular belief; rather, they carry handguns they bring from home (Center for the Prevention of
Handgun Violence, 1991).

Although the issue of gun control is quite controversial,
we must seriously explore ways to keep guns from the hands
of children and adolescents. A recent article by Christoffel
(1991) examines a number of strategies, ranging from a
handgun ban to holding adults responsible for a minor's use
of a gun that the adult has not properly secured.

In addition to restricting youth's access to guns, children need to be taught that guns are dangerous. One attempt in this area is a curriculum designed by the Center for
the Prevention of Handgun Violence (1991) for children in
kindergarten through 12th grade. Noting that children are
taught the potential dangers of matches and electrical out-
lets, but not guns, the curriculum uses exercises and facts
about violence with guns to instruct children on the lethality
of weapons. For example, one such exercise involved older
children doing an analysis of a *Time* magazine article ("Seven
Deadly Days," 1989) that pictured a week's homicide victims
along with the circumstances of each murder. The purposes
of the exercise were to give these youth an appreciation of
the circumstances of homicide (usually expressive), and to
dispel the myth that most people are killed by strangers in
the commission of a crime.

Strengthening of Racial Identity

There is some evidence that strong ethnic identity may decrease involvement in self-destructive behaviors (Gary and Berry, 1985). At the least, a sense of ethnic pride and respect should lead to greater value's being attached to, for example, African-American life; as a result, involvement in activities that destroy that life should decrease, and involvement in activities and institutions that support and enhance that life should increase.

Using the African-American experience as a model, African-American professionals and business people are sponsoring programs geared toward helping the least fortunate and most vulnerable in the African-American community. For example, several years ago the president of an African-American hair care company in Chicago established the Black-on-Black Love Campaign, which was aimed at creating respect for self and for other African-Americans. As part of the campaign, the company adopted a building in a public housing development and invested in a library, a computer lab, a ceramics shop, and an outdoor mural exhibiting African-American pride. According to the police, since this program has been in place there have been decreased gang activity, fewer fights, and less graffiti on the walls of this building.

Other examples of such activities are "mentor" programs, in which a youth is "adopted" by a nonfamily member who serves as a role model and provides practical support. These activities are usually undertaken by organizations or ad hoc groups that work through schools and community organizations. Such programs for male adolescents may involve "manhood initiation rites" that enhance the youth's sense of racial identity and communal responsibility.

The long-term impact of these programs on violence and aggression has yet to be assessed. However, one study found that African-American students in an Afrocentric curriculum (Devarics, 1990) showed a rise in grades and self-esteem, suggesting the importance of these values and activities.

Secondary Prevention

"Secondary prevention" refers to measures that can be taken before the problem does damage that is irreversible. In terms of homicide, this means identifying and treating perpetrators and victims of nonlethal violence, as well as intervening in the violence process before it results in a death.

Identification and Treatment of Victims and Perpetrators

One of the most obvious places for identifying and treating violence and potentially violent youngsters is the juvenile justice system. In general, youngsters who have already committed a violent but nonlethal act should be considered at risk for committing more serious violence (Lewis et al., 1985). Such youngsters can be ordered by the courts to receive treatment. Currently, the National Commission on Correctional Health Care, the accrediting body for the health care components of the criminal justice system, is planning an intervention program in the nation's juvenile detention centers that will focus on identifying and intervening with violence-prone youth before the youngsters seriously hurt someone; this program is described in more detail below.

Just as violent behavior is viewed as an indicator of the potential for more serious violence, being a victim is also related to the perpetration of violence. That is, consistent with findings on adults (Wolfgang, 1958; Singer, 1986), youthful offenders and victims have similar characteristics (Jensen and Bronsonfield, 1986), with perpetrators having a history of victimization (McDermott, 1983; Uehara et al., in press). As noted earlier, such findings point out that these youth live in a violent milieu in which the roles of victim and perpetrator alternate. The research shows that this similarity between victims and perpetrators is not present in elementary school children; aggressors and instigating bystanders of elementary age have different attitudes and problem-solving strategies than do victims (Guerra and Slaby, 1990). It also demonstrates that identification of and intervention with victims are important in breaking up the violence cycle, particularly as some research indicates that victimization leads to perpetration (Uehara et al., in press).

The notion that homicide is a public health issue, not a criminal justice one, does not mean that the police do not have a role in its reduction. Indeed, the police are often the first to become aware of assault victims and perpetrators, and are ideally situated for identifying and referring for treatment those individuals at risk for homicide. Hospital emergency rooms are also a prime source of identification and referral of persons at risk. Furthermore, it is suggested that physicians, clinics, and health care facilities routinely screen for patients' involvement in violence (Bell et al., 1988a, 1988b) and make referrals where appropriate. Protocols for identifying, as well as treating, victims of interpersonal violence are available and have been shown to work in emergency rooms, where such patients are frequently found (*Report of the Surgeon General's Workshop on Violence and Public Health,* 1986).

Current research at the Community Mental Health Council, Inc. (CMHC) is being supported by the United Way of Chicago in order to identify the prototype for a comprehensive emergency room interpersonal violence intervention service, as well as gaps in current services in Cook County. Elements of a comprehensive service that have already been identified are protocols for identifying and treating victims; the ability to refer battered women to shelters; proper evidence collection and documentation for possible legal action; the ability to refer victims to support groups and help them to obtain victims' compensation aid; the ability to refer perpetrators and violent families for treatment; the potential to generate policy changes designed to reduce variables that increase the risk of violence; outreach and follow-up components; collaboration with local law enforcement; and of course appropriate medical treatment for injuries. The last factor is often taken for granted, but it may well be that the decrease in homicides that was starting in 1986 (Griffith and Bell, 1989) was attributable in part to the sophistication of trauma care by hospital emergency room trauma networks. With the advent of faster-firing and more lethal weapons (McKinley, 1990; Fountain and Recktenwald, 1990), and the gradual deterioration of trauma networks in poor communities where such care is the most needed, the more recent increases in homicide may also be in part attributable to a decrease in the number of nonlethal gunshot wounds.

Gynecologists can routinely inquire about their patients' involvement in domestic violence and, at the least, make available handbooks on domestic violence. Victimization screening of the mentally ill is especially encouraged, as this group is at increased risk for assault (Bell et al., 1988b) and homicide (Hillard et al., 1985); their victimization has important implications for their treatment. The need for routine screenings is important, as research indicates that individuals often will not give unsolicited information regarding an incident but will respond honestly if asked directly (Jacobson et al., 1987). Also, routine screening for violence exposure, along with other physical and mental health problems, legitimizes it as a health problem that can be treated.

As previously mentioned, victims (both adults [Wolfgang, 1958; Singer, 1986] and youth [McDermott, 1983]) often have a history of perpetration, and some evidence indicates that victimization predicts perpetration among youth (Uehara et al., in press). Thus, since both victims and perpetrators can be referred for psychological services when identified by agencies with which they come into contact, screening in public schools can identify victims and potential perpetrators—or, at the least, youngsters who need to address their feelings and possible trauma in regard to victimization (Shakoor and Chalmers, 1991). The Violence Prevention Project in Boston has pediatric nurses doing follow-up with adolescents and their families who come to the city hospital with intentional injuries (Wilson-Brewer et al., 1990). Juvenile detention centers are also obvious places to screen for adolescent victims or witnesses of violence, as well as obvious places to conduct violence prevention workshops and/or provide counseling to violence-prone youth.

The National Commission on Correctional Health Care (1991) is planning an intervention for violence among youth that is similar to its efforts to address the issue of AIDS prevention in juvenile detention facilities. Because the commission is an accrediting body for health care components of jails, prisons, and juvenile detention facilities, it is in an excellent position to help establish disease or intentional injury prevention programs in such facilities, where high-risk youth are found. Recognizing the fact that juveniles in detention facilities were at high risk for contracting HIV infection, the commission developed a manual for health care workers in juvenile correctional facilities to use in teaching youth about AIDS and ways to keep from getting HIV-infected. Next, they had a national training conference for health care professionals in those facilities; finally, they are providing local technical assistance in getting this prevention program up and running in juvenile facilities. This same model of intervention is now being implemented in regard to issues of victimization, management of violence in facilities, and conflict resolution (National Commission on Correctional Health Care, 1991).

Screening for victimization may be a necessary step in various types of primary prevention programs, such as those described above. Clearly, the application of violence prevention methods will need to be very different, depending on whether an individual has or has not been a victim, perpetrator, or witness of violence. Regardless of the way in which youthful victims, perpetrators, and witnesses are identified, steps must be taken to make sure that appropriate and adequate services are available to them (Spivak et al., 1987; Bell and Jenkins, 1990). Many mental health centers do not provide programs for adult victims and offenders, let alone for youthful ones. In this regard the article by Pynoos and Nader (1988) is very useful, as it outlines psychologic first aid for children exposed to community violence. This article lists the symptomatic responses to such violence shown by children at different developmental stages, and describes procedures for assisting these children that are specific to their level of development.

Individuals working with these groups may require special training and/or selection, as they will need expertise in the treatment of victims and young offenders. An understanding of childhood and adolescent development and an appreciation of the milieu in which the youngsters function are essential. As is often the case when working with violent individuals, the counselors must be sensitive to negative transference and countertransference.

Intervening in Violent Situations

In general, few people who work with children and adolescents know how to intervene in violent or potentially violent situations in a manner that de-escalates the violence, short of overpowering the involved parties. Fewer still know how to respond in truly dangerous situations, such as a shooting or sniper incident. As the Illinois State Police (1989) noted in developing their school security program, for example, school officials know how to handle a fire, but there are few policies that describe what to do if a student brings a gun to school.

The Illinois State Police (1989) school security program recommends strategies for preventing and handling violence in schools, and emphasizes how to recognize volatile individuals and situations before they get out of hand. Specific tactics vary by level of severity of violence, ranging from potentially violent individuals and situations to situations that require physical intervention.

Being able to handle violent situations, even life-threatening ones, in the school is critical, as the number of shootings in and near schools is becoming distressingly frequent. Under these circumstances, school personnel must secure their environment—not only so that they can teach and the children can learn, but so that children can have at least one safe haven from the violence that often permeates their lives. In many situations, neighborhood violence is rampant, and children often witness violence in the home as well; thus, these children have no place in their lives where they can feel safe. The extent to which children witness and are aware of violence in their neighborhoods and homes is not to be underestimated. Such violence exposure has a serious impact on the children's mental health and is a risk factor in the perpetration of violence.

Tertiary Prevention

Tertiary prevention occurs after considerable damage has been done. Unfortunately, in the case of homicide, it refers to interventions that occur after a murder has been committed. Although the death cannot be reversed, the morbidity of family members and friends of the homicide victims (and perpetrators) may be significant and demands that these "covictims" be serviced by health professionals and social support systems. Being family members or friends of a person who was murdered, particularly in a grisly manner, often predisposes these individuals to feelings of grief, stress, and depression, and possibly to post-traumatic stress disorder (PTSD) and major depression (Rynearson, 1986).

Services for Those Exposed to Homicide

As one would expect from the high homicide rate, exposure to homicide—as a witness and/or as a friend or relative of a victim—is extensive. In a CMHC survey of its clients, 25% reported that someone close to them had been murdered (Bell et al., 1988b); 29% of a medical outpatient group had had a "significant other" murdered (Bell et al., 1988a). Distressingly, this knowledge and exposure are not limited to adults. In Los Angeles and Detroit, it has been estimated that between 10% and 20% of all murders are witnessed by a dependent youngster (Pynoos and Eth, 1985; Batchelor and Wicks, 1985). A CMHC survey of 536 elementary school children found that one-quarter had seen someone shot (Jenkins and Thompson, 1986); a survey of 1,000 high school students found that 23% had seen someone killed, and that 40% of those victims were family, friends, classmates, or neighbors (Shakoor and Chalmers, 1991).

Being exposed to, and especially witnessing, homicide can lead to a number of emotional problems associated with PTSD, including depression and anxiety, impaired cognitive functioning (with direct implications for learning and achievement—see below), and an increase in aggression and behavioral problems (Pynoos and Eth, 1985). In one study of male students referred from the same classroom for behavior problems and poor academic performance, all of them had an extensive history of family violence resulting in the murder of at least one family member (Dyson, 1990). Dyson noted that unresolved grief for these losses was a major factor in the boys' acting out and aggressive behavior. One elementary school in south central Los Angeles had so many students experiencing violence and death of significant others that a regular class was instituted to address issues of grief and loss (Timnick, 1989).

These clinical observations indicate that youthful witnesses/covictims of homicide may have a variety of behavioral or psychological problems. Youth who have witnessed the murder of a parent (Pynoos and Eth, 1985), or who are exposed to lethal community violence (Pynoos and Nader, 1990), may have classic symptoms of PTSD. They may recreate the traumatic incident in their play, have dreams of the incident, or have the traumatic memory intrude in their daily lives. They may develop psychic numbing, indicated by passivity, decreased motor behavior, inactivity, diminished range of affect, and a bland, uninterested style of life. Clinical evidence of sleep disorders, avoidance behaviors, and fearfulness may also be present. Fears of the event's recurring; guilt over their not having been able to intervene in the incident; a foreshortened sense of their own future, with a resulting nihilistic perspective and risk-taking behaviors; and difficulty in establishing relationships—all these may result from the psychological trauma of experiencing lethal violence. Youth exposed to deadly violence may also have low-ered self-esteem (Hyman et al., 1988). In addition, problems in school performance may occur as the result of fatigue from sleepless nights and traumatic memories' intruding and distracting from learning; a cognitive style involving memory lapses may develop, which, while protecting the psyche, in-terferes with learning (Pynoos and Nader, 1988). The specif-ic symptoms that a given youth may develop will depend on that youth's personality, age, and developmental level, as well as other buffering influences in the youth's life, such as family support. On the one hand, there may be a tendency to self-destructive behaviors such as aggressiveness, substance abuse, delinquency, or promiscuity. On the other hand, the youth may take a pseudo-self-sufficient stance with an at-tempt at premature entry into adulthood, in an effort to escape the risk factors associated with adolescence.

It is essential to recognize the psychological aftermath of homicide for witnesses and survivors and to provide appropriate services. It is equally essential to come to grips with the reality that many people, particularly inner-city children, exist in what can only be described as war zones; even if they physically survive the chronic threats they ex-perience, these threats will seriously diminish their life chances by blighting their cognitive and emotional develop-ment. Given the pervasiveness of the problem, it is important that high-risk areas be routinely screened for exposure to deadly violence by school personnel, and that appropriate services be instituted in the schools (Shakoor and Chalmers, 1991).

As noted above in connection with secondary preven-tion, Pynoos and Nader (1988) have outlined methods of delivering psychologic first aid to children who witness com-munity violence. The interventions for youth who are sub-jected to the traumatic stress of violence depend on their developmental status and age. Adolescents, for example, are prone to engage in fantasies about retaliation and revenge, and these notions can be explored and addressed in an effort to reduce the impetus for actualizing the ideas or taking out violent urges on an innocent bystander.

Since one review has found no significant correlation between the exposure to lethal violence (as either a covictim or a witness) and later perpetration of violence (Widom, 1989), considerable research needs to be done on factors that mediate the impact of exposure to such violence (Bell and Jenkins, 1991). Factors that have been proposed to buffer the impact of being exposed to deadly violence include development of conflict resolution skills; the development of a strong ethnic identity; a strong extended family network, with multiple caregivers available; the subject's socioeconomic status or class; spiritual development; rural versus urban background; developmental age during the exposure; whether the victim was a stranger or an intimate; single or chronic exposure to violence; the response of the child's milieu toward the violent incident; education; whether the violence was expressive or instrumental; whether the violence was "rational" or "irrational"; and innate constitutional factors of the person who was exposed. Such knowledge could be a firm basis for future interventions.

Services for Perpetrators

Although service providers may be reluctant to deal with perpetrators of homicide because of negative transference, individuals who commit murder and are released back into the community (usually through parole) need treatment, particularly if they are suffering from neuropsychiatric impairment. Often these individuals need aid in coping with their impulsive act of homicide, in readjusting to the community, or in managing a chronic mental illness.

Juveniles who have already perpetrated deadly violence are at higher risk of (again) committing such violence than nonviolent youth. In view of this, it seems only reasonable to address the myriad issues relating to the previous violent behaviors in an effort to prevent future violence. To this end, the treatment efforts directed toward a youth who has committed a homicide will very closely resemble the treatment efforts discussed above in regard to youth who perpetrate nonlethal violence. Thus, the same exploration of the youth's previous experiences with violence and victimization, the emphasis on strengthening nonviolent conflict resolution skills, the provision of violence-free environments, and so forth are all indicated in treating youthful perpetrators of homicide.

SUMMARY

Knowledge and research in the area of youth violence and homicide are just beginning to move beyond the understanding that intentional injury is a public health problem with various implications for treatment and prevention. The basic questions of the epidemiology of violence/homicide and the prevalence of exposure to violence/homicide are beginning to be answered. This process now raises even more complicated questions regarding mediating factors and consequences, as well as possible prevention and intervention strategies. Issues of nihilism, risk-taking behaviors, willingness to form close relationships, the development of dissociative states of consciousness, and a lack of strong future orientation are all currently being explored with regard to youth violence and homicide. Finally, the need to evaluate prevention and intervention measures more carefully is recognized, as it is essential that proposed methods of correcting the problem be efficacious and replicable. Given the seriousness and pervasiveness of the problem of youth violence/homicide, many different groups (government, education, public health, law enforcement, mental health, private sector, church, etc.) must work together to mount a multifaceted public health approach to eliminating or at least alleviating it.

CHAPTER NINE

Epilogue

Chapter 9 consists of three sections. The first section summarizes the major findings of the book, followed by a brief discussion of various issues in adolescence, such as cognition and gender, that are related to suicide and homicide among youth. The second section focuses specifically on demographic issues in the prevention and intervention of youth suicide and homicide; primary, secondary, and tertiary prevention are discussed. The third section synthesizes prevention and intervention strategies: From all the reviews, programs, and levels of conceptualization for preventing and intervening in youth suicide and homicide, four common strategies emerge: (1) gun control, (2) public education, (3) training of professionals, and (4) research. The first two strategies are primarily epidemiologic in nature, the third is more clinical, and the fourth includes both epidemiologic and clinical perspectives.

SUICIDE, HOMICIDE, AND THE ADOLESCENT

Summary of Our Major Findings

In this book, youth suicide and homicide have been studied from epidemiologic and clinical perspectives. Emphasis has been placed on the importance of utilizing both these viewpoints and their interactions to obtain a more complete picture of youth suicide and homicide.

Youth suicide and homicide account for 30% of all deaths among adolescents and young adults (i.e., youth aged 15–24) in the United States. There are both similarities and differences in the epidemiologic patterns of suicide and homicide among youth. The similarities are the patterns over time (period effects), with the rates being higher in the 1930s, lower in the 1940s and 1950s, increasing in the 1960s and 1970s, and, recently, tending toward a decrease in the rate of rise (among 15- to 19-year-olds) and a leveling off (among 20- to 24-year-olds); the numerical rates themselves, current rates being close to or at their highest levels since data collection for the entire United States began in 1933; the increase of rates with age throughout adolescence and young adulthood; and the gender pattern, with male rates being higher than female rates for all age and race groups. The differences between the epidemiologic patterns of youth suicide and homicide are primarily in the ethnic area: For suicide, rates for white males are greater than for nonwhite males, whereas for homicide, rates for nonwhite males are far greater than for white males.

It is important, however, to remind ourselves that counting numbers of suicides and homicides has only been done for the entire United States since 1933. Data from before that date are incomplete and less reliable. Data from before 1900 are almost nonexistent. In addition, the mass media now report most homicides and suicides among the young. The average citizen is therefore much more aware of what type of violent behavior takes place in his or her society than in previous generations. The overall violent death rate is lower now than in the early 1900s (Holinger, 1987), and, if anything, we believe that rates of violent death among youth today are probably lower than in previous centuries. We say this because life in the past seems to have been cheaper, and young people were perhaps more at the mercy of their elders (e.g., witness the prior existence of child sacrifice, child slavery, and child labor). In contrast to the first half of this century, there have been no major world wars in the past 50 years, or nearly two generations. In this context, we might take exception with the common view that the violence shown in movies and on TV is responsible to some extent for actual violence. Rather, it may be that this movie and TV violence is a manifestation of our greater capacity to understand our internal frustrations and violence, and to symbolize and represent them visually and auditorially. This idea would be consistent with the decrease of violent death rates and wars over the century.

Cross-cultural studies show that U.S. youth suicide rates fall approximately in the upper third of rates for various countries, but that the youth homicide rates in the United States are far higher than in nearly any other country. Economic and demographic variables may be related to the long-term increase and decrease in youth suicide and homicide and to nonmortality measures of psychopathology among youth; the importance of these variables lies in the potential for prediction and intervention.

Although epidemiologic similarities exist between youth suicide and homicide, important clinical differences exist as well. Youth who commit suicide are characterized by major psychiatric problems: major affective disorders (bipolar disorder or major depression), schizophrenia, character disorder, or a combination of these. Comorbidity of these disturbances with substance abuse appears to be particularly lethal. Youth homicide most often involves poverty and the apparently related interpersonal, domestic, and gang-related violence; victims and perpetrators share similar characteristics. Character disorders (e.g., impulse control, sociopathic problems) appear common to both victims and perpetrators of youth homicide. Treatment of suicidal youth includes psychotherapy, pharmacotherapy, family therapy, and hospitalization. For youth homicide, various primary, secondary, and tertiary strategies have been outlined for potential victims and perpetrators, with an emphasis on intervening at various levels of the domestic violence cycle. The apparent clinical differences between youth suicide and homicide may be a result of the greater level of sophistication found currently in the suicide studies.

Cognitive Abilities and Gender Differences

Recent findings suggest that adolescence is characterized by the emergence of new mental capacities that allow adolescents to consider possibilities and alternatives more fully

(Keating, 1990). The thought process is definitely no longer child-like. Adolescents are now able to think in sophisticated ways about their social and interpersonal world. This change in adolescents' cognitive abilities includes an increased complexity in their conceptions about mental illness, which in turn influence their willingness to participate in treatment. That is, Piaget's theory of cognitive development would also suggest that adolescents may be more capable of the kind of hypothetical–deductive reasoning necessary for reflecting about possible courses of action for seeking help. In addition, these more sophisticated cognitive abilities should allow the adolescents the opportunity to benefit from psychotherapeutic interventions. It should be noted, however, that these growing cognitive abilities have been hypothesized to contribute to the depression and social withdrawal of adolescents with disabilities (Elkind, 1985). Elkind posits that these new mental constructions give adolescents the ability "to reconstruct their childhood and to see it in a very different light from the way they perceived [it] as children" (p. 84). Elkind suggests that these new capabilities can exacerbate existing disabilities. These newly acquired abilities also make it more possible for adolescents to plan and execute a suicide or a homicide.

Yet, at the same time that adolescents become able to engage successfully in violent behavior, they still appear to retain a relatively child-like conception of death. It is only slowly that they learn to appreciate the finality of death. This might explain why adolescents engage in considerably more risky behavior than adults (Arnett, personal communication, 1993). The freedom with which adolescents so often seem to engage in dangerous behavior may be related to their belief that they (as well as their friends) are invulnerable. Risky behavior is not necessarily related to mental illness; that is, an adolescent does not have to suffer from a psychiatric syndrome (e.g., bipolar disorder or schizophrenia) in order to behave dangerously. Along similar lines, it seems to us that some adolescents make a serious suicide attempt with a belief that they will still wake up the next morning. These suicide attempts are not always made with deep commitment to a wish to die. In like fashion, an adolescent who has killed another often seems genuinely amazed that the adolescent who was shot is actually dead; hence the rationale of one homicide prevention program which involves taking adolescent gang members to the morgue to see the bodies of their dead friends or enemies. The same sense of invulnerability is also seen in homicide—the teenager who blithely walks through a neighborhood controlled by an unfriendly gang, or the youngster who threatens an obviously dangerous peer, daring the peer to fight. These last examples involve adolescents whose risky behavior may result to some extent from both an inadequate conceptualization of death and an inability to channel aggression in more socially acceptable ways.

As we have noted throughout the book, youth suicide and homicide both show marked gender differences, and a complex interaction of factors appears to account for this. For example, gender differences in social-cognitive ability exist in adolescence. It appears that emotionally disturbed adolescent girls score higher than boys on measures assessing different aspects of social-cognitive ability, such as moral reasoning (Schonert, 1992) and ego development (Paget et al., 1990). Other research has indicated that females in general score higher in domains theoretically related to social-cognitive ability, such as empathy (Hoffman, 1977), altruism (Krebs, 1975), and the decoding of visual and auditory cues (Hall, 1978). Thus, adolescent girls may be better able than adolescent boys to benefit from insight-oriented treatment approaches. Adolescent girls in general can make better use of their social field to help them vent frustration and unhappiness. Their social skills serve as an excellent buffer, allowing many girls to verbalize their feelings without acting on them. In contrast, boys are by nature more action-oriented; they often cope by "doing something about it." We have found that for both homicide and suicide the rates for young males are considerably and consistently higher than those for young females—sometimes three to four times higher.

We suggest that even to this date, the culture's expectations for the male (in ancient times, the hunter or gatherer) differ from those for the female (in ancient times, the caretaker). In this sense, both the poor African-American adolescent male and his white middle-class male peer who die a violent death are those who on some level believe that they cannot, for whatever reason, fulfill the role expected of them. This can also be seen as a failure of the social order, in that it does not present enough flexibility to its youth as they grow up and attempt to find a place within the society. The adolescent female, despite the considerable pressure that has been placed on her in the United States in the last decade, still has more options than boys as she grows up to adulthood. Therefore, she may not be as desperate as often as her male peer—and hence the female suicide and homicide rates are considerably lower than the male rates. It is our prediction, however, that as women become truly equal to men in the labor force, with expectations similar to those for men, the rates of suicide and homicide for females will become more like those of men.

DEMOGRAPHIC ISSUES IN PREVENTION AND INTERVENTION

Throughout this book, we have suggested that one useful way to explore youth suicide and homicide is via the clinical–epidemiologic interaction—that is, by examining internal vulnerability (e.g., biologic or characterologic disorders) in combination with external stresses (e.g., social forces such as economic and demographic variables). Durkheim was the person most responsible for establishing the systematic study of the relationships between social forces and suicide. His major study, *Suicide: A Study in Sociology* (1897/1951), has become a classic in sociology as well as suicidology. Durkheim appeared to view society and its impact in at least two different ways. The first was in terms of delineated groups (e.g, religions), and one of Durkheim's categories of suicide, "altruistic suicide," involved this concept. It referred more to a consciously or preconsciously delineated group, and consisted of taking one's own life because of greater integration of the individual into society (e.g., religious affiliation or unthinking political allegiance). His second concept of society was more complex and leaned more toward Easterlin's and Brenner's subsequent ideas of social forces. For example, two of Durkheim's categories of suicide, "egoistic suicide" and "anomic suicide," demonstrate the concept of social forces driving suicide rates. However, Durkheim went even further than Brenner and Easterlin in positing social factors as the key influence in shifts in suicide rates. Durkheim tended to minimize the intrapsychic, rather than to attempt to build bridges between intrapsychic and societal factors. For instance, he suggested that suicide rates are high in times of economic stress because the social cohesion of the group is broken down. He did not attempt to detail on an individual level how this may occur, as Brenner and Easterlin have done.

Although much work has been performed on the impact of economic variables on suicide and homicide trends, far less has been done on the impact of demographic variables. This section examines the issues of intervention and prevention with reference to demography. Of all the variables associated with youth suicide and homicide, only the demographic ones are able to predict long-term patterns. We use the categories of primary, secondary, and tertiary prevention here, because the demographic perspective creates special opportunities in these areas.

Primary Prevention

Educational Institutions

There are a number of possible preventive strategies involving high schools and colleges. First, the educational institutions need to be aware of the fluctuating populations of young people. This is especially true during times of increase, as occurred from the mid-1950s to the late 1970s, and as will occur during the late 1990s. There often exists a lag time in society's response to such an increase in population, and this lag time needs to be shortened. For educational institutions, this means expanding enrollment facilities, dorms, faculties, and so forth at the beginning of the increase, not afterward. With an increased number of adolescents will come an increased number of psychologically vulnerable youth who are at risk—and this risk will be increased if more and more teenagers who want to go to college cannot do so because of space limitations.

Within the educational institutions themselves, the work of Barker and Gump (1964) and Barker (1968) posits that smaller schools, in which students are actively involved in extracurricular activities, athletics, and so on, provide an atmosphere that better enhances the students' sense of well-being. Psychologically, it appears that those smaller schools are better able to provide external sources of self-esteem and attention, which can be critical in aiding psychologically vulnerable, at-risk youth as they mature. Various implications for both large and small educational institutions arise from these findings. For example, during periods of increase in the number of adolescents, it would appear essential to increase the numbers of athletic teams to allow fuller participation, and to enlarge the varieties of extracurricular programs as well as the size of existing activities. In addition, the numbers of academic programs and honors should be increased. For example, instead of just one first-place prize in a certain subject, second- and third-place honors might also be included. These issues are discussed further below.

Two other issues with respect to educational institutions need to be considered: classes and counseling services. The content of the classes would be psychologic and would include studies of affects, descriptions of depression, and clinical clues about youthful suicide and homicide. Of all the things children are taught, it is essential that some understanding of affects be conveyed. As we have noted throughout, there has been an explosion in research in infant development during the past decade (e.g., Stern, 1985; Basch, 1988), and much has been learned about human beings and their emotional development. This information should be used to aid youth in labeling, understanding, and communicating their feelings; such an endeavor seems worthy of study with respect to the possible impact on suicide and homicide rates. Similarly, teaching material on depression and signs of self-destructive tendencies among youth might also be effective in decreasing rates, although there is recent controversy on this issue (e.g., Shaffer and Bacon, 1989). Educators might also consider making such a class available to, or even mandatory for, parents of teenagers. On the larger scene, such classes would be valuable for younger children and their parents; such information should be disseminated through the schools or, for parents, through pediatricians and obstetricians.

With respect to counseling in the educational institutions, two issues emerge: the availability of counselors and the screening of students. More high school and college counselors are needed, and they need to be well trained in the areas of depression, domestic violence, suicide, and homicide. Another idea regarding availability is a "hotline" telephone system specifically directed at teenagers, who could call if depressed, suicidal, involved in domestic violence, or the like. Miller et al. (1984) demonstrated a decrease in suicide rates among young women in areas that had suicide prevention facilities. In addition, there is the possibility that an annual or twice-a-year screening of adolescents might help in decreasing the suicide and homicide rates during periods of increased numbers of youth. Such screening might consist of a brief pencil-and-paper screening test assessing depression, suicidal ideation, domestic violence, and so on. An annual screening of this type seems worthy of further study (e.g., Yufit, 1989).

The Business Community

The business community also has a role in decreasing suicide and homicide rates during periods of increased numbers of adolescents. It is now well documented that increased unemployment is associated with an increase in suicide and homicide rates (Brenner, 1971, 1979). In addition, an unusually large cohort of youth may flood the business market and cause an increase in unemployment in that age group, with an associated rise in suicide and homicide rates (Easterlin, l980). What appears necessary is an increased awareness on the part of the business community of these associations and of the periods of increasing numbers of youth. Efficacious responses on the part of business would include increasing youthful employment during these periods of increasing teenage population, not only during summer months but year-round as well.

Secondary Prevention

Secondary prevention relates to intervention and is particularly concerned with suicide attempts and domestic violence. The health care delivery system is the most involved at the level of secondary prevention. With an increasing number of adolescents, the health care system becomes overloaded with depressed teenagers, adolescent suicide attempters, abused teenagers, and so on; psychiatrists, psychologists, and psychiatric social workers are too busy and are not able to take new patients or see them soon enough; outpatient clinics are too full or do not respond as quickly as necessary; and hospital emergency rooms are too overburdened and relatively understaffed to adequately identify and treat depressed, suicidal, or abused youngsters. An awareness of the issue is important at the governmental, hospital, and practitioner levels. For example, the government will need to fund additional training of psychiatrists and other mental health professionals, particularly in the area of adolescent psychiatry. Hospitals and schools need to adjust appropriately their staffing and facilities to handle this increase in patients.

Tertiary Prevention

Tertiary prevention, or postvention, is aimed at decreasing psychopathology in family members, friends, and schools following a suicide or homicide. Of particular recent concern is the controversial question of whether or not suicide clusters and "contagion" exist—that is, whether one or two suicides among youth influence further suicides and suicide attempts. The various issues and interventions in such circumstances are well documented (e.g., see CDC, 1988a). The question here is to what extent such clusters and contagions are influenced by increasing numbers of youth. It appears that the government, school systems, communities, parents, and youth need to be aware of this potential danger during times of large youthful cohorts, with attention to appropriate interventions during those periods.

Many of the interventions noted above have not been adequately researched and tested in terms of their potential for decreasing suicide and homicide rates. At least three strategies suggest themselves. The first is a before-and-after strategy. Communities, school systems, and the like could be compared with respect to their suicide and homicide rates before and after various adjustments were made; of course, the possibility of a variety of confounding variables would have to be kept in mind. Second, various schools and school systems could be compared with respect to suicide and homicide rates. The variables might include size (large vs. small), demographic areas, and so on, or might involve specific interventions (e.g., schools that taught classes in affects and recognition of depression and domestic violence could be compared with schools that did not). Finally, within individual schools, studies are needed on a variety of interventions: screening of students; increases in activities, athletic teams, and honors; and relevant classes on affect, depression, and domestic violence. Such comparative studies within individual schools would involve a variety of strategies (e.g., half the students could participate in an intervention and the other half could serve as a control group; the use of interventions could be alternated by grades; etc.).

PREVENTION AND INTERVENTION STRATEGIES: A SYNTHESIS

The epidemiologic and clinical factors discussed throughout this book should dictate intervention and prevention strategies. There are marked similarities and differences in the etiologies of youth suicide and homicide, and there are a wide variety of conceptualizations of intervention and prevention. With respect to reducing suicide and homicide among youth, a comprehensive and integrated approach seems crucial: Variables such as child development issues, poverty and jobs, firearm access, training of professionals, teaching conflict resolution skills, and so forth, must all be considered. Yet, as we attempt to organize and synthesize these approaches, four major issues stand out:

1. *Gun control.* The availability of guns must be limited if any significant decrease in youthful suicide and homicide is to be achieved. The accumulating data no longer allow ambivalence on this issue (e.g., Zimring, 1991; Móscicki and Boyd, 1983–1985; Brent et al., 1991; Rosenberg et al., 1991; Sloan et al., 1990; Kassirer, 1991; Loftin et al., 1991; Cotton, 1992; Marzuk et al., 1992b; *Journal of the American Medical Association,* 1992).

2. *Public education.* Enough is now known about the etiologies of suicide and homicide among youth to warrant massive public attention to these issues. Effective treatment and prevention strategies exist, and the public should be informed about them.

3. *Training of professionals.* Professionals in fields related to suicide and homicide among youth need to be better trained. In the case of suicide, this means physicians, social workers, and various counseling professionals, as well as teachers, clergy, and so on. For homicide, training should include the police, as well as others potentially involved in situations of domestic violence (e.g., emergency room doctors, teachers, clergy, etc.) (Council on Ethical and Judicial Affairs, 1992; Sugg and Inui, 1992).

4. *Research.* Despite the major studies over the past decade, more knowledge of etiology and treatment is needed, both epidemiologic and clinical. Such increased knowledge is especially critical with respect to the characterologic and biologic aspects of the victims and perpetrators of homicide.

Suicide Rates for 15- to 19-Year-Olds, by Sex and Race, United States, 1933–1990

Year	Total	White males	White females	Nonwhite males	Nonwhite females
1933	4.1	4.7	3.9	2.7	3.0
1934	4.4	4.9	4.3	3.7	2.5
1935	4.2	4.8	4.1	2.5	1.6
1936	4.2	5.3	3.4	3.8	2.6
1937	3.9	5.0	3.3	2.8	1.7
1938	4.1	5.2	3.5	3.1	1.6
1939	3.7	4.8	3.0	1.7	1.6
1940	3.5	4.3	3.0	3.0	1.8
1941	3.4	4.3	3.0	1.8	2.1
1942	3.1	4.0	2.4	2.1	2.1
1943	3.1	4.2	2.3	2.8	1.0
1944	2.8	3.7	2.4	1.7	1.3
1945	2.8	4.4	1.9	2.0	0.3
1946	3.0	4.1	2.3	1.6	1.9
1947	3.0	4.2	1.9	2.8	2.2
1948	2.8	3.8	2.2	1.2	0.6
1949	2.5	3.8	1.5	2.4	0.9
1950	2.7	3.7	1.9	2.2	1.5
1951	2.6	3.8	1.7	1.8	1.7
1952	2.9	4.7	1.4	1.9	0.8
1953	2.8	4.2	1.8	1.6	1.8

(continued)

Sources of data: See Figure 1.1.

Year	Total	White males	White females	Nonwhite males	Nonwhite females
1954	2.4	3.5	1.2	1.7	1.8
1955	2.6	4.0	1.4	4.0	1.0
1956	2.3	3.5	1.2	2.5	1.8
1957	2.5	4.1	1.0	3.3	0.7
1958	3.0	4.7	1.8	1.4	0.8
1959	3.4	5.4	1.6	3.4	1.7
1960	3.6	5.9	1.6	3.4	1.5
1961	3.4	5.5	1.6	3.7	1.3
1962	3.8	5.6	1.9	3.6	1.9
1963	4.0	6.2	1.9	3.6	2.0
1964	4.0	6.7	1.7	4.0	1.8
1965	4.0	6.3	1.9	5.2	2.4
1966	4.3	6.7	2.1	4.8	2.4
1967	4.7	7.5	2.5	3.8	3.5
1968	5.1	8.3	2.2	4.7	2.2
1969	5.7	9.0	2.6	5.8	3.2
1970	5.9	9.4	2.9	5.4	3.0
1971	6.5	10.4	3.0	6.1	3.6
1972	6.9	11.1	2.7	5.5	3.4
1973	7.0	11.4	3.2	6.8	2.7
1974	7.2	11.9	3.3	6.3	2.8
1975	7.6	13.1	3.1	7.0	2.2
1976	7.4	11.9	3.3	8.4	2.5
1977	8.9	15.3	3.5	8.1	2.4
1978	8.0	13.8	3.4	7.5	1.6
1979	8.6	14.6	3.4	8.9	2.4
1980	8.5	15.0	3.3	7.5	1.8
1981	8.7	14.9	3.9	7.2	2.2
1982	8.7	15.5	3.4	7.2	1.9
1983	8.7	15.1	3.5	8.7	2.1
1984	9.0	15.8	3.8	7.3	2.3
1985	10.0	17.3	4.1	10.0	2.2
1986	10.2	18.2	4.1	8.0	2.5
1987	10.3	17.6	4.4	9.9	2.9
1988	11.3	19.6	4.8	11.0	2.6
1989	11.3	19.4	4.5	12.1	3.1
1990	11.1	19.3	4.0	13.0	2.5

Homicide Rates for 15- to 19-Year-Olds, by Sex and Race, United States, 1933–1990

Year	Total	White males	White females	Nonwhite males	Nonwhite females
1933	6.7	4.8	2.2	49.8	15.2
1934	6.1	4.5	1.8	43.6	16.1
1935	5.4	3.4	2.1	41.9	12.9
1936	4.8	3.0	1.7	33.3	16.5
1937	5.4	3.3	2.0	42.4	13.8
1938	4.7	2.5	1.6	37.4	14.3
1939	4.4	2.3	1.0	38.1	14.8
1940	4.0	2.0	0.8	35.7	14.8
1941	4.2	2.1	1.0	35.6	16.1
1942	4.4	2.6	0.9	34.6	15.4
1943	4.1	2.4	1.1	36.9	8.7
1944	3.7	2.4	0.8	32.4	7.8
1945	4.5	3.2	0.9	36.7	11.4
1946	4.0	2.9	1.1	29.9	9.7
1947	3.9	2.2	0.9	33.1	10.1
1948	4.1	2.2	1.0	37.1	9.5
1949	4.0	2.6	1.1	30.3	9.7
1950	3.9	2.6	1.2	27.5	10.7
1951	3.7	2.2	1.0	29.8	9.6
1952	4.2	2.4	1.1	34.7	9.1
1953	3.6	2.2	1.0	29.6	6.7

(*continued*)

Sources of data: See Figure 1.1.

195

Year	Total	White males	White females	Nonwhite males	Nonwhite females
1954	3.7	2.3	1.3	28.2	7.2
1955	3.2	2.3	0.8	22.9	7.3
1956	3.5	2.3	1.2	23.6	8.3
1957	3.7	2.3	1.3	26.9	6.9
1958	3.8	2.8	1.3	26.0	7.9
1959	3.6	2.7	1.1	23.3	8.6
1960	4.1	3.2	1.2	27.6	7.0
1961	3.6	2.7	1.1	25.9	6.0
1962	3.7	2.5	1.3	26.5	6.2
1963	3.6	2.8	1.0	24.5	6.1
1964	4.3	2.9	1.4	30.9	7.7
1965	4.3	3.0	1.3	30.8	7.1
1966	5.1	3.4	1.6	38.0	7.9
1967	6.1	4.3	1.6	43.8	9.3
1968	6.9	5.1	1.6	49.6	9.6
1969	7.8	4.9	1.9	59.7	11.0
1970	8.1	5.2	2.1	60.2	10.1
1971	8.5	5.5	2.1	60.2	13.0
1972	8.8	6.4	2.8	61.4	13.5
1973	9.1	7.1	3.1	51.5	13.1
1974	9.8	7.8	3.2	54.2	14.0
1975	9.6	8.2	3.2	47.8	14.6
1976	8.6	7.5	3.0	43.2	10.5
1977	9.0	8.3	3.1	40.9	12.3
1978	8.9	8.7	3.5	37.1	10.3
1979	10.5	10.7	3.7	43.6	11.7
1980	10.6	10.9	3.9	43.3	10.1
1981	10.2	10.0	3.5	43.0	9.7
1982	9.8	9.2	3.5	41.7	10.1
1983	8.5	7.6	2.9	37.3	9.7
1984	8.3	7.5	3.2	34.3	9.0
1985	8.6	7.3	2.7	39.9	9.4
1986	10.0	8.6	3.3	44.2	10.8
1987	10.0	7.3	3.0	50.3	10.5
1988	11.7	8.1	3.0	64.4	10.2
1989	13.7	9.6	3.3	75.7	10.0
1990	17.0	12.5	3.6	92.0	12.8

Suicide Rates for 20- to 24-Year-Olds, by Sex and Race, United States, 1933–1990

Year	Total	White males	White females	Nonwhite males	Nonwhite females
1933	10.5	13.9	8.0	9.4	5.0
1934	10.5	14.7	7.1	9.1	6.2
1935	10.2	14.6	6.7	7.9	5.8
1936	9.5	13.3	6.8	7.4	3.4
1937	10.1	14.5	6.9	6.3	5.1
1938	9.5	14.0	5.8	5.2	4.3
1939	8.3	12.5	4.9	6.4	3.9
1940	8.9	13.6	4.9	7.6	4.8
1941	8.1	11.6	5.3	8.9	3.0
1942	7.1	10.8	4.1	8.3	3.6
1943	6.1	9.0	4.1	7.4	2.2
1944	6.1	9.6	4.1	6.9	2.7
1945	7.0	12.7	4.0	9.7	4.1
1946	7.3	11.0	4.3	8.5	2.8
1947	6.2	9.3	3.5	7.4	3.1
1948	6.6	9.8	3.8	8.6	2.0
1949	6.5	9.9	3.7	6.8	2.4
1950	6.2	9.4	3.5	8.4	1.9
1951	6.1	9.7	2.9	9.0	3.2
1952	5.6	9.2	2.7	7.4	1.8
1953	6.0	10.0	2.9	7.5	2.2

(continued)

Sources of data: See Figure 1.1.

Year	Total	White males	White females	Nonwhite males	Nonwhite females
1954	6.0	10.3	2.4	10.1	1.3
1955	5.6	8.7	2.6	9.5	2.7
1956	5.9	9.6	2.8	9.6	0.6
1957	5.8	9.4	2.7	8.5	2.1
1958	7.0	11.2	3.1	10.4	2.8
1959	6.8	11.0	2.8	10.6	2.9
1960	7.1	12.0	3.1	7.8	1.6
1961	7.1	10.9	3.2	12.5	2.9
1962	8.2	12.2	4.0	12.2	4.2
1963	8.5	12.5	4.4	12.2	3.1
1964	8.4	12.8	4.4	13.5	2.3
1965	8.9	13.9	4.3	13.1	4.0
1966	9.2	14.2	4.5	14.1	3.6
1967	9.7	14.9	4.8	14.4	4.7
1968	9.6	15.1	4.8	13.1	4.4
1969	10.7	17.0	5.0	15.4	5.2
1970	12.3	19.3	5.7	19.4	5.5
1971	12.5	19.0	6.2	17.8	7.1
1972	14.0	20.6	6.6	26.0	8.2
1973	14.8	24.3	5.5	23.3	5.8
1974	15.1	24.5	6.4	21.3	5.0
1975	16.5	26.8	6.9	23.6	6.0
1976	16.4	27.0	6.6	22.6	5.7
1977	18.6	30.8	7.5	24.3	5.8
1978	16.9	28.1	6.7	23.3	5.0
1979	16.9	27.5	6.7	25.4	5.5
1980	16.2	27.8	5.9	20.9	3.6
1981	15.6	26.9	5.9	18.4	3.8
1982	15.1	26.5	5.4	17.6	3.9
1983	14.8	25.5	5.5	17.8	3.8
1984	15.6	27.5	5.5	18.4	3.5
1985	15.6	27.4	5.2	20.2	3.5
1986	15.8	28.4	5.3	17.5	2.9
1987	15.3	27.5	4.7	19.0	3.1
1988	15.0	27.0	4.4	20.0	3.0
1989	15.3	26.8	4.3	24.1	3.9
1990	15.1	26.8	4.4	20.6	3.0

Homicide Rates for 20- to 24-Year-Olds, by Sex and Race, United States, 1933–1990

Year	Total	White males	White females	Nonwhite males	Nonwhite females
1933	16.0	12.1	3.9	132.6	31.9
1934	16.9	12.5	3.9	146.3	31.4
1935	14.2	10.2	3.6	121.7	28.9
1936	13.7	9.7	3.2	113.8	34.7
1937	13.6	8.5	3.2	124.6	33.9
1938	11.7	7.7	3.1	102.7	28.2
1939	10.6	6.4	1.4	105.7	31.3
1940	10.4	5.9	1.8	105.5	28.4
1941	10.2	5.3	2.0	107.4	28.2
1942	9.6	5.2	1.5	99.3	28.7
1943	7.9	4.9	1.4	77.0	21.5
1944	7.9	5.5	1.3	81.1	22.0
1945	9.6	7.8	1.9	98.6	22.0
1946	10.7	7.2	2.1	97.2	27.2
1947	10.2	6.2	1.7	102.2	24.3
1948	9.9	6.0	2.0	96.4	23.2
1949	9.1	5.3	1.7	87.1	24.5
1950	8.5	4.7	1.4	86.4	20.6
1951	8.0	5.0	1.5	75.8	20.8
1952	8.2	5.4	1.7	80.5	17.2
1953	8.4	5.6	1.4	82.8	17.6

(*continued*)

Sources of data: See Figure 1.1.

Year	Total	White males	White females	Nonwhite males	Nonwhite females
1954	8.4	5.8	1.6	75.6	18.0
1955	8.0	4.9	1.7	71.3	17.5
1956	8.9	6.0	1.7	78.2	18.0
1957	8.2	5.7	1.5	69.0	17.6
1958	8.2	5.5	1.9	67.1	17.6
1959	8.6	6.0	1.8	73.1	16.8
1960	8.2	6.0	1.9	64.1	16.4
1961	8.2	5.5	2.0	67.3	16.1
1962	8.7	5.4	2.1	74.0	16.3
1963	8.6	5.7	1.8	70.3	16.2
1964	8.8	6.4	1.7	74.9	15.6
1965	10.0	7.4	2.3	80.5	17.3
1966	10.9	7.2	2.5	94.4	18.8
1967	12.7	8.7	2.9	105.8	24.7
1968	14.0	10.6	2.8	115.4	24.5
1969	14.9	10.9	3.0	126.1	21.7
1970	16.0	11.1	3.5	136.4	23.9
1971	17.2	12.1	3.0	150.7	23.6
1972	18.8	13.2	3.2	152.7	28.9
1973	18.4	14.4	4.5	128.2	27.8
1974	19.2	15.5	4.4	131.7	18.2
1975	18.3	14.5	4.8	124.9	23.7
1976	16.6	13.9	4.2	103.4	24.3
1977	16.6	14.9	4.7	94.8	22.0
1978	17.6	16.3	4.7	99.7	22.3
1979	19.3	18.9	5.2	101.2	23.4
1980	20.6	19.9	5.5	109.4	23.3
1981	18.9	18.5	5.0	95.5	21.2
1982	17.3	16.7	5.3	84.6	17.1
1983	15.8	15.1	4.4	78.0	18.0
1984	15.3	14.3	5.2	71.2	16.9
1985	15.1	14.6	4.3	72.8	15.2
1986	17.9	16.0	5.1	91.0	18.0
1987	17.8	14.8	4.7	92.9	20.3
1988	19.0	14.8	4.7	105.6	19.7
1989	20.0	15.7	4.4	113.4	19.6
1990	22.5	18.1	4.5	126.8	18.1

References

Ambrosini PJ, Rabinovich H, Puig-Antich J. Biological factors and pharmacologic treatment in major depressive disorder in children and adolescents. In *Suicide in the Young* (Sudak HS, Ford AB, Rushforth NB, eds.). Boston: John Wright/PSG, 1984.

American School Health Association. *National Adolescent Student Health Survey*. Washington, DC: American School Health Association, Association for the Advancement of Health Education, Society for Public Health Education, 1988.

Anthony EJ. Two contrasting types of adolescent depression and their treatment. *Journal of the American Psychoanalytic Association* 18:841–859, 1970.

Aro HM, Marttunen MJ, Lönnqvist JK: Trends in suicide mortality among young people in Finland. *Psychiatrica Fennica* 23:29–39, 1992.

Barker RG. *Ecological Psychology*. Stanford, CA: Stanford University Press, 1968.

Barker RG, Gump PV. *Big School, Small School: High School Size and Student Behavior*. Stanford, CA: Stanford University Press, 1964.

Baron JN, Reiss PC. Reply to Phillips and Bollen. *American Sociological Review* 50:372–376, 1985.

Barrett TW, Scott TB. Suicide bereavement and recovery patterns compared with nonsuicide bereavement patterns. *Suicide and Life-Threatening Behavior* 20:1–15, 1990.

Basch MF. *Understanding Psychotherapy: The Science behind the Art*. New York: Basic Books, 1988.

Batchelor J, Wicks N. *Study of Children and Youth as Witness to Homicide, city of Detroit*. Detroit: Family Bereavement Center, Frank Murphy Hall of Justice—Victim Services, 1985.

Bell CC. Coma and the etiology of violence, Part I. *Journal of the National Medical Association* 78:1167–1176, 1986.

Bell CC. Coma and the etiology of violence, Part II. *Journal of the National Medical Association* 79:79–85, 1987.

Bell CC, Hildreth CJ, Jenkins EJ, Carter C. The need for victimization screening in a poor, outpatient medical population. *Journal of the National Medical Association* 80:853–860, 1988a.

Bell CC, Jenkins EJ. Preventing black homicide. In *The State of Black America—1990* (Dewart J, ed.). New York: National Urban League, 1990.

Bell CC, Jenkins EJ. Traumatic stress and children. *Journal of Health Care for the Poor and Underserved* 2(1):175–188, 1991.

Bell CC, Taylor-Crawford K, Jenkins EJ, Chalmers D. Need for victimization screening in a black psychiatric population. *Journal of the National Medical Association* 80:41–48, 1988b.

Benedek EP, Cornell DG. *Juvenile Homicide*. Washington, DC: American Psychiatric Press, 1989.

Berman AL. Fictional depiction of suicide in television film and imitation effects. *American Journal of Psychiatry* 145:982–986, 1988.

Block CR. *Homicide in Chicago*. Urban Insights Series No. 14. Chicago: Loyola University of Chicago, Center for Urban Policy, 1986.

Block CR. Lethal violence in the Chicago Latino community. In *Homicide: The Victim/Offender Interaction* (Wilson AV, ed.). Cincinnati: Anderson, 1993.

Blumenthal SJ, Kupfer DJ. Overview of early detection and treatment strategies for suicidal behavior in young people. *Journal of Youth and Adolescence* 17:1–23, 1988.

Braungart RG, Braungart MM. Youth status and national development: A global assessment in the 1980's. *Journal of Youth and Adolescence* 18:107–130, 1989.

Brenner MH. *Time Series Analysis of Relationships between Selected Economic and Social Indicators*. Springfield, VA: National Technical Information Service, 1971.

Brenner MH. *Mental Illness and the Economy*. Cambridge, MA: Harvard University Press, 1973.

Brenner MH. Mortality and the national economy. *Lancet* ii:568–573, 1979.

Brent DA, Perper JA, Allman CJ, Moritz GM, Wartella ME, Zelenak JP. The presence and accessibility of firearms in the homes of adolescent suicides: A case–control study. *Journal of the American Medical Association* 266:2989–2995, 1991.

Brent DA, Perper JA, Goldstein CE, Kolko DJ, Allan MJ, Allman

CJ, Zelenak JP. Risk factors for adolescent suicide. *Archives of General Psychiatry* 45:581–588, 1988.

Brooke EM. *Suicide and Attempted Suicide.* Public Health Papers No. 58. Geneva, Switzerland: World Health Organization, 1974.

Busch KG, Zagar R, Hughes JR, Arbit J, Bussell RE. Adolescents who kill. *Journal of Clinical Psychology* 46:472–489, 1990.

Cain AC (ed.). *Survivors of Suicide.* Springfield, IL: Charles C Thomas, 1972.

Campbell M, Perry R, Green WH. Use of lithium in children and adolescents. *Psychosomatics* 25:95–105, 1984.

Campbell M, Spencer E. Psychopharmacology in child and adolescent psychiatry: A review of the past 5 years. *Journal of the American Academy of Child and Adolescent Psychiatry* 27:269–279, 1988.

Cantor P. The effects of youthful suicide on the family. *Psychiatric Opinion* 12:6–11, 1975.

Center for the Prevention of Handgun Violence. *Straight Talk about Risks.* Washington, DC: Center for the Prevention of Handgun Violence, 1991.

Centers for Disease Control (CDC). *Homicide Surveillance: High-Risk Racial and Ethnic Groups—Blacks and Hispanics, 1970 to 1983.* Atlanta: Centers for Disease Control, November 1986.

Centers for Disease Control (CDC). Recommendations for a community plan for the prevention and containment of suicide clusters. *Morbidity and Mortality Weekly Reports* 37(Suppl. S-6):1–11, 1988a.

Centers for Disease Control (CDC). Premature mortality due to homicides: United States, 1968–1985. *Morbidity and Mortality Weekly Reports* 37:543–545, 1988b.

Centers for Disease Control (CDC). Weapon-carrying among high-school students—United States, 1990. *Morbidity and Mortality Weekly Reports* 40:681–684, 1991.

Chemtob CM, Hamada RS, Gauer G, Kinney B, Torigoe RY. Patients' suicides: Frequency and impact on psychiatrists. *American Journal of Psychiatry* 145:224–228, 1988.

Christoffel KK. Violent death and injury in U.S. children and adolescents. *American Journal of Diseases of Children* 144:697–706, 1990.

Christoffel KK. Toward reducing pediatric injuries from firearms: Charting a legislative and regulatory course. *Pediatrics* 88:294–305, 1991.

Clark D. Combination murder–suicide. *Suicide Research Digest* 4(4):12,14, 1990.

Classification of Terms and Comparability of Titles through Five Revisions of the International List of Causes of Death. Vital Statistics—Special Reports, Vol. 19, No. 13. Washington, DC: U.S. Department of Commerce, Bureau of the Census, 1944.

Comer J. *School Power: Implications of an Intervention Project.* New York: Free Press, 1980.

Comer J. Educating poor minority children. *Scientific American* 259:42–48, 1988a.

Comer J. *Maggie's American Dream.* New York: New American Library, 1988b.

Corrigan PW, Yudofsky SC, Silver JM. Pharmacological and behavioral treatments for aggressive psychiatric inpatients. *Hospital and Community Psychiatry* 44:125–133, 1993.

Cotton P. Gun-associated violence increasingly viewed as public health challenge. *Journal of the American Medical Association* 267:1171–1174, 1992.

Council of Ethical and Judicial Affairs, American Medical Association. Physicians and domestic violence: Ethical considerations. *Journal of the American Medical Association* 267:3190–3193, 1992.

Cullberg J, Wasserman D, Stafansson C.-G. Who commits suicide after a suicide attempt? An 8 to 10 year follow up in a suburban catchment area. *Acta Psychiatrica Scandinavica* 77:598–603, 1988.

Dahlgren KG. *On Suicide and Attempted Suicide.* Lund, Sweden: A.-B. PH. Lindstedts Univ.-Bokhandel, 1945.

Davidson L, Gould MS. Contagion as a risk factor for youth suicide. In *Report of the Secretary's Task Force on Youth Suicide. Vol. 2: Risk Factors For Youth Suicide.* DHHS Pub. No. (ADM) 89–1622. Washington, DC: U.S. Government Printing Office, 1989.

Death Rates by Age, Race, and Sex, United States, 1900–1953: Selected Causes. Vital Statistics—Special Reports, Vol. 43. Washington, DC: U.S. Department of Commerce, Bureau of the Census, 1956.

Dennis RE, Kirk A, Knuckles BN. *Black Males at Risk for Low Life Expectancy: A Study of Homicide Victims and Perpetrators.* Washington, DC: National Institute of Mental Health, Center for Studies of Minority Group Mental Health, 1981.

Devarics C. Afro-centric program yields academic gains. *Black Issues in Higher Education* 7:1–34, 1990.

Diekstra RFW. Suicide, depression and economic conditions. In

Current Concepts of Suicide (Lester D, ed.). Philadelphia: Charles Press, 1990.

Dodge KA. A social information processing model of social competence in children. In *Minnesota Symposium on Child Psychology*, Vol. 18 (Perlmutter M., ed.). Hillsdale, NJ: Erlbaum, 1986.

Dorpat TL, Ripley HS. A study of suicide in the Seattle area. *Comprehensive Psychiatry* 1:349–359, 1960.

Dunn HL, Shackley W. *Comparison of Cause-of-Death Assignments by the 1929 and 1938 Revisions of the International List: Deaths in the United States, 1940.* Washington, DC: U.S. Department Commerce, Bureau of the Census, Vital Statistics—Special Reports, Vol. 19, No. 14. 1944.

Durkheim E. *Suicide: A Study in Sociology* (Spaulding JA, Simpson G, Trans.). Glencoe, IL: Free Press, 1951. (Original work published 1897)

Dyson J. The effects of family violence on children's academic performance and behavior. *Journal of the National Medical Association* 82:17–22, 1990.

Earls F. Studying adolescent suicidal ideation and behavior in primary care settings. *Suicide and Life-Threatening Behavior* 19:99–107.

Easterlin RA. *Birth and Fortune.* New York: Basic Books, 1980.

Elkind D. Cognitive development and adolescent disabilities. *Journal of Adolescent Health Care* 6:84–89, 1985.

Ettlinger RW. Suicides in a group of patients who had previously attempted suicide. *Acta Psychiatrica Scandinavica* 40:363–378, 1964.

Ewing CP. *When Children Kill: Dynamics of Juvenile Homicide.* Lexington, MA: Lexington Books, 1990.

Farberow NL. Preparatory and prior suicidal behavioral factors. In *Report of the Secretary's Task Force on Youth Suicide. Vol. 2: Risk Factors for Youth Suicide.* DHHS Pub. No. (ADM) 89-1622. Washington, DC: U.S. Government Printing Office, 1989.

Faust MM, Dolman AB. *Comparability of Mortality Statistics for the Fifth and Sixth Revisions: United States, 1950.* Vital Statistics—Special Reports, Vol. 51, No. 2. Washington, DC: U.S. Department of Commerce, Bureau of the Census, 1963.

Faust MM, Dolman AB. *Comparability Ratios Based on Mortality Statistics for the Fifth and Sixth Revisions: United States, 1950.* Vital Statistics—Special Reports, Vol. 51, No. 3. Washington, DC: U.S. Department of Commerce, Bureau of the Census, 1964.

Faust MM, Dolman AB. *Comparability of Mortality Statistics for the Sixth and Seventh Revisions: United States, 1958.* Vital Statistics—Special Reports, Vol. 51, No. 4. Washington, DC: U.S. Department of Commerce, Bureau of the Census, 1965.

Fingerhut LA, Kleinman JC. International and interstate comparisons of homicide among young males. *Journal of the American Medical Association* 263:3292–3295, 1990.

Fingerhut LA, Kleinman JC, Godfrey E, Rosenberg H. *Firearm Mortality among Children, Youth, Adults, 1–34 years of age, Trends and Current Status: United States, 1979–88.* Monthly Vital Statistics Report, Vol. 39, No. 11, Suppl. Hyattsville, MD: U.S. Public Health Service, 1991.

Flango VE, Sherbonou EL. Poverty, urbanization, and crime. *Criminology* 14:331–346, 1976.

Fountain JW, Recktenwald W. One youth's death sums up '90 summer. *Chicago Tribune*, Section 1, pp. 1 and 11, September 24, 1990.

Fowler RC, Rich CL, Young D. San Diego Suicide Study: II. Substance abuse in young cases. *Archives of General Psychiatry* 43:962–968, 1986.

Freiberg P. Killing by kids "epidemic" forecast. *American Psychological Association Monitor* pp. 1 and 31, April 1991.

Freud S. Mourning and melancholia. *Standard Edition* (London: Hogarth Press) 14:237–258, 1957. (Original work published 1917)

Furst J, Huffine CL. Assessing vulnerability to suicide. *Suicide and Life-Threatening Behavior* 21:329–344, 1991.

Garrison CZ, Lewinsohn PM, Marstellar F, Langhinrichsen J, Lann I. The assessment of suicidal behavior in adolescents. *Suicide and Life-Threatening Behavior* 21:217–230, 1991.

Gary LE, Berry GL. Predicting attitudes toward substance abuse in a black community: Implications for prevention. *Community Mental Health Journal* 21:42–51, 1985.

Gelles R. *The Violent Home.* Newbury Park, CA: Sage, 1987.

Gist R, Welsh QB. Certification change versus actual behavior changes in teenage suicide rates, 1955–1979. *Suicide and Life-Threatening Behavior* 19:277–287, 1989.

Goldberg A. *The Prisonhouse of Psychoanalysis.* Hillsdale, NJ: Analytic Press, 1990.

Goldney RD, Katsikitis M. Cohort analysis of suicide rates in Australia. *Archives of General Psychiatry* 40:71–74, 1983.

Goodman RA, Mercy JA, Loya F, Rosenberg ML, Smith JC, Allen

NH, Vargas L, Kolts R. Alcohol use and interpersonal violence: Alcohol detected in homicide victims. *American Journal of Public Health* 76:144–149, 1986.

Goodwin FK, Brown GL. Summary and overview of risk factors in suicide. In *Report of the Secretary's Task Force on Youth Suicide. Vol 2: Risk Factors for Youth Suicide.* DHHS Pub. No. (ADM) 89-1622. Washington, DC: U.S. Government Printing Office, 1989.

Gordon RE, Gordon KK. Social psychiatry of a mobile suburb. *International Journal of Social Psychiatry* 6:89–106, 1960.

Gould MS, Shaffer D. The impact of suicide in television movies. *New England Journal of Medicine* 315:690–694, 1986.

Gould MS, Wallenstein S, Kleinman M. *A Study of Time–Space Clustering of Suicide: Final Report.* Contract No. RFP 200-85-0834. Atlanta: Centers for Disease Control, 1987.

Griffith EEH, Bell CC. Recent trends in suicide and homicide among blacks. *Journal of the American Medical Association* 262:2265–2269, 1989.

Guerra NG, Slaby RG. Cognitive mediators of aggression in adolescent offenders: 2. Intervention. *Developmental Psychology* 26:269–277, 1990.

Haim A. *Adolescent Suicide* (Smith AMS, trans.). New York: International Universities Press, 1974.

Hall JA. Gender effects in decoding nonverbal cues. *Psychological Bulletin* 85:845–858, 1978.

Hammond WR, Yung BR. *Dealing with Anger.* Champaign, IL: Research Press, 1991.

Hanzlick R, Gowitt GT: Cocaine metabolite detection in homicide victims. *Journal of the American Medical Association* 265:760–761, 1991.

Hawkins DF. Black and white homicide differentials: Alternatives to an inadequate theory. In *Homicide among Black Americans* (Hawkins DF, ed.). Lanham, MD: University Press of America, 1986.

Hendin H. *Suicide in America.* New York: Norton, 1982.

Hendin H. Psychodynamics of suicide, with particular reference to the young. *American Journal of Psychiatry* 148:1150–1158, 1991a.

Hendin H. Trauma of losing loved one to suicide is similar to PTSD. *The Psychiatric Times,* p. 59, November 1991b.

Henry AF, Short JF. *Suicide and Homicide: Some Economic, Sociological and Psychological Aspects of Aggression.* Glencoe, IL: Free Press, 1954.

Herzog A, Levy L, Verdonk A. Some ecological factors associated with health and social adaptation in the city of Rotterdam. *Urban Ecology* 2:205–234, 1977.

Hillard JR, Slomowitz M, Levi LS. A retrospective study of adolescent visits to a general hospital psychiatric emergency service. *American Journal of Psychiatry* 145:1416–1419, 1987.

Hillard JR, Zung W, Ramm D. Accidental and homicide death in a psychiatric emergency room population. *Journal of Hospital and Community Psychiatry* 36:640–642, 1985.

Hoffman ML. Sex differences in empathy and related behaviors. *Psychological Bulletin* 84:712–722, 1977.

Holford TR. The estimation of age, period and cohort effects for vital rates. *Biometrics* 39:1311–1324, 1983.

Holinger PC. Adolescent suicide: An epidemiologic study of recent trends. *American Journal of Psychiatry* 135:754–756, 1978.

Holinger PC. Violent deaths as a leading cause of mortality: An epidemiologic study of suicide, homicide, and accidents. *American Journal of Psychiatry* 137:472–476, 1980.

Holinger PC. *Violent Deaths in the United States: An Epidemiologic Study of Suicide, Homicide, and Accidents.* New York: The Guilford Press, 1987.

Holinger PC. The causes, impact, and preventability of childhood injuries in the United States: Childhood suicide in the United States. *American Journal of Diseases of Children* 144:670–676, 1990a.

Holinger PC. The impact of developmental psychology and infant research on psychotherapy and psychoanalysis. *Directions in Psychiatry* 10(23):1–8, 1990b.

Holinger PC, Holinger DP, Sandlow J. Violent deaths among children in the United States, 1900–1980: An epidemiologic study of suicide, homicide, and accidental deaths among 5–14 year olds. *Pediatrician: International Journal of Child and Adolescent Health* 12:11–19, 1983–1985.

Holinger PC, Klemen EH. Violent deaths in the United States, 1900–1975. *Social Science and Medicine* 16:1929–1938, 1982.

Holinger PC, Lester D. Suicide, homicide, and demographic shifts: An epidemiologic study of regional and national trends. *Journal of Nervous and Mental Disease* 179:574–575, 1991.

Holinger PC, Offer D. Perspectives on suicide in adolescence. In *Social and Community Mental Health*, Vol. 2 (Simmons R, ed.). Greenwich, CT: JAI Press, 1981.

Holinger PC, Offer D. Prediction of adolescent suicide: A population model. *American Journal of Psychiatry* 139:302–307, 1982.

Holinger PC, Offer D. Toward the prediction of violent deaths among the young. In *Suicide in the Young* (Sudak HS, Ford AB, Rushforth NB, eds.). Boston: John Wright/PSG, 1984.

Holinger PC, Offer D. The epidemiology of suicide, homicide, and accidents among adolescents, 1900–1980: Trends and potential prediction. In *Advances in Adolescent Mental Health* (Feldman R, Stiffman A, eds.). Greenwich, CT: JAI Press, 1986.

Holinger PC, Offer D. Sociodemographic, epidemiologic, and individual attributes. In *Report of the Secretary's Task Force on Youth Suicide. Vol. 2: Risk Factors for Youth Suicide.* DHHS Pub. No. (ADM) 89-1622. Washington, DC: U.S. Government Printing Office, 1989.

Holinger PC, Offer D, Ostrov E. Suicide and homicide in the United States: An epidemiologic study of violent death, population changes, and the potential for prediction. *American Journal of Psychiatry* 144:215–219, 1987.

Holinger PC, Offer D, Zola M. A prediction model of suicide among youth. *Journal of Nervous and Mental Disease* 176:275–279, 1988.

Hurry A. My ambition is to be dead. *Journal of Child Psychotherapy* 4:66–83, 1977.

Hurry A. Past and current findings on suicide in adolescence. *Journal of Child Psychotherapy* 4:69–82, 1978.

Hyman IA, Zelikoff W, Clark J. Psychological and physical abuse in schools: A paradigm for understanding post-traumatic stress disorder in children and youth. *Journal of Traumatic Stress* 1:243–267, 1988.

Illinois State Police. *School Security Program.* Springfield: Illinois State Police, 1989.

Institute of Medicine, National Academy of Science. *Injury in America.* Washington, DC: National Academy Press, 1985a.

Institute of Medicine, National Academy of Sciences. *Discussion Summary from Workshop on Forecasting Stress-Related Social Problems.* Washington, DC: National Academy of Sciences, Division of Mental Health and Behavioral Medicine, September 26–27, 1985b.

Jacobson A, Koehler JE, Jones-Brown C. The failure of routine assessment to detect histories of assault experienced by psychiatric patients. *Hospital and Community Psychiatry* 38:386–389, 1987.

Jenkins EJ, Bell CC. Adolescent violence: Can it be curbed? *Adolescent Medicine: State of the Art Reviews* 3(1):71–86, 1992.

Jenkins EJ, Thompson B. Children talk about violence: Preliminary findings from a survey of black elementary school children. Paper presented at the 19th Annual Convention of the Association of Black Psychologists, Oakland, CA, 1986.

Jensen GF, Bronsonfield D. Gender, lifestyles and victimization: Beyond routine activity. *Violence and Victims* 1:85–99, 1986.

Johnston LD, O'Malley PM, Bachman JG. *Smoking, Drinking, and Illicit Drug Use among Secondary Students, College Students, and Young Adults, 1975–1991. Vol. 1: Secondary School Students.* Rockville, MD: U.S. Department of Health and Human Services, National Institute on Drug Abuse, 1992.

Journal of the American Medical Association 267(22), June 10, 1992.

Judson DS. Research proposal. Unpublished manuscript, 1993.

Kassirer J. Firearms and the killing threshold. *New England Journal of Medicine* 325:1647–1650, 1991.

Kavka J. The suicide of Richard Cory: An explication of the poem by Edward Arlington Robinson. *Annual of Psychoanalysis* 4:479–500.

Keating D. Adolescent thinking. In *At the Threshold: The Developing Adolescent* (Feldman SS, Elliott GR, eds.). Cambridge, MA: Harvard University Press, 1990.

Kellerman AL, Reay DT. Protection or peril?: An analysis of firearm-related deaths in the home. *New England Journal of Medicine* 314:1557–1560, 1986.

Kernberg PF. *Borderline Conditions and Pathological Narcissism.* New York: Jason Aronson, 1975.

Kernberg PF. The analysis of a 15½ year old girl with suicidal tendencies. In *The Analyst and the Adolescent at Work* (Harley M, ed.). New York: Quadrangle, 1974.

Kessler RC, Downey G, Milavsky JR, Stipp H. Clustering of teen-age suicides after television news stories about suicides. *American Journal of Psychiatry* 145:1379–1383, 1988.

Kessler RC, Stipp H. The impact of fictional television stories on U.S. fatalities. *American Journal of Sociology* 90:151–167, 1984.

Klebba AJ. Homicide trends in the United States, 1900–1974. *Public Health Reports* 90:195–204, 1975.

Klebba AJ. Comparison trends for suicide and homicide in the United States, 1900–1976. In *Violence and the Violent Individual* (Hays JR, ed.). New York: SP Medical & Scientific Books, 1979.

Klebba AJ, Dolman AB. *Comparability of Mortality Statistics for the Seventh and Eighth Revisions of the International Classification of Diseases, United States.* Vital Health Statistics, Vol. 2, No. 66. Washington, DC: U.S. Government Printing Office, 1975.

Klerman G. The current age of youthful melancholia. *British Journal of Psychiatry* 152:4–14, 1988.

Klerman G. Suicide, depression, and related problems among the baby boom cohort. In *Suicide among Youth: Perspectives on Risk and Prevention* (Pfeffer CR, ed.). Washington, DC: American Psychiatric Press, 1989.

Klerman GL, Lavori PW, Rice J. Birth-cohort trends in rates of major depressive disorder among relatives of patients with affective disorder. *Archives of General Psychiatry* 42:689–693, 1985.

Klerman GL, Weissman MM. An epidemiologic view of mental illness, mental health, and normality. In *Normality and the Life Cycle: A Critical Integration* (Offer D, Sabshin M, eds.). New York: Basic Books, 1984.

Kohut H. *The Analysis of the Self.* New York: International Universities Press, 1971.

Kohut H. *How Does Analysis Cure?* Chicago: University of Chicago Press, 1984.

Kotlowitz A. Urban trauma: Day-to-day violence takes a terrible toll on inner-city youth. *The Wall Street Journal,* pp. 1, 26, October 27, 1987.

Kotlowitz A. *There Are No Children Here.* New York: Doubleday, 1991.

Kovacs M, Puig-Antich J. "Major psychiatric disorders" as risk factors in youth suicide. In *Report of the Secretary's Task Force on Youth Suicide. Vol. 2: Risk Factors for Youth Suicide.* DHHS Pub. No. (ADM) 89-1622. Washington, DC: U.S. Government Printing Office, 1989.

Kramer M, Pollack ES, Redick RW, Locke BZ. *Mental Disorders/ Suicide.* Cambridge, MA: Harvard University Press, 1972.

Krebs D. Empathy and altruism. *Journal of Personality and Social Psychology* 32:1124–1146, 1975.

Lalonde M. *A New Perspective on the Health of Canadians.* Ottawa: Tri-Graphic Printing, 1974.

Lann IS, Mościcki EK, Maris R (eds.). Special issue: Strategies for studying suicide and suicidal behavior. *Suicide and Life-Threatening Behavior* 19:1–146, 1989.

Laufer M. The analysis of an adolescent at risk: With comments on the relation between psychopathology and technique. In *The Analyst and the Adolescent at Work* (Harley M, ed.). New York: Quadrangle, 1974.

Levy JC, Deykin EY. Suicidality, depression and substance abuse in adolescence. *American Journal of Psychiatry* 146:1462–1467, 1989.

Levy L, Herzog A. Effects of population density and crowding on health and social adaptation in the Netherlands. *Journal of Health and Social Behavior* 15:228–240, 1974.

Levy L, Herzog A. Effects of crowding on health and social adaptation in the city of Chicago. *Urban Ecology* 3:327–354, 1978.

Lewis DO, Moy E, Jackson RD, Aaronson R, Restifo N, Serra S, Simos A. Biopsychosocial characteristics of children who later murder: A prospective study. *American Journal of Psychiatry* 142:1161–1167, 1985.

Linehan MM. Suicidal people: One population or two? *Annals of the New York Academy of Sciences* 487:16–33, 1986.

Litman RE. Psychological autopsies of youth suicides. In *Report of the Secretary's Task Force on Youth Suicide. Vol. 3: Prevention and Interventions in Youth Suicide.* DHHS Pub. No. (ADM) 89-1623. Washington, DC: U.S. Government Printing Office, 1989.

Litman RE, Curphey T, Shneidman ES, Farberow NL, Tabachnick N. Investigations of equivocal suicides. *Journal of the American Medical Association* 184:924–929, 1963.

Litt I, Cuskey W, Rudd S. Emergency room evaluation of the adolescent who attempts suicide: Compliance with follow-up. *Journal of Adolescent Health Care* 4:106–108, 1983.

Loftin C, Hill RH. Regional subculture and homicide: An examination of the Gastil–Hackney thesis. *American Sociological Review* 39:714–724, 1974.

Loftin C, McDowall D, Wiersema B, Cottey TJ. Effects of restrictive licensing of handguns on homicide and suicide in the District of Columbia. *New England Journal of Medicine* 325:1615–1620, 1991.

MacDonald JM. *The Murderer and His Victim.* Springfield, IL: Charles C Thomas, 1961.

MacMahon B, Pugh TF. *Epidemiology: Principles and Methods.* Boston: Little, Brown, 1970.

Males M. Teen suicide and changing cause of death certification, 1953–1987. *Suicide and Life-Threatening Behavior* 21:245–259, 1991.

Maltsberger JT, Buie DH. Countertransference late in the treatment of suicidal patients. *Archives of General Psychiatry* 30:625–633, 1974.

Marzuk PM, Leon AC, Tardiff K, Morgan EB, Stojic M, Mann JJ. The effect of access to lethal methods of injury on suicide rates. *Archives of General Psychiatry* 49:451–458, 1992b.

Marzuk PM, Tardiff K, Hirsch CS. The epidemiology of murder–suicide. *Journal of the American Medical Association* 267:3179–3183, 1992a.

McDermott J. Crime in the school and in the community: Offenders, victims, and fearful youth. *Crime and Delinquency* 29:270–282, 1983.

McKinley JC. The new dealers' guns: More bullets, going faster. *New York Times*, Section B, p. 3, August 1, 1990.

Miller HC, Coombs DW, Leeper JD, Burton SN. An analysis of the effects of suicide prevention facilities in the United States. *American Journal of Public Health* 74:340–343, 1984.

Miller LS. *Murder in Illinois: 1973–1982.* Springfield: Illinois Criminal Justice Information Authority, 1983.

Mościcki EK, Boyd JH. Epidemiologic trends in firearm suicides among adolescents. *Pediatrician: International Journal of Child and Adolescent Health* 12:52–62, 1983–1985.

Mościcki EK, O'Carroll PW, Rae DS, Roy AG, Locke BZ, Regier DA. Suicidal ideation and attempts: The Epidemiologic Catchment Area study. In *Report of the Secretary's Task Force on Youth Suicide. Vol. 4: Strategies for Prevention of Youth Suicide.* DHHS Pub. No. (ADM) 89-1624. Washington, DC: U.S. Government Printing Office, 1989.

Motto J. Suicide attempts: A longitudinal view. *Archives of General Psychiatry* 13:516–520, 1965.

Murphy E, Lindesay J, Grundy E. Sixty years of suicide in England and Wales. *Archives of General Psychiatry* 43:969–977, 1986.

Murphy GE. Suicide and attempted suicide. In *The Medical Basis of Psychiatry.* (Winokur G, Clayton P, eds.). Philadelphia: W.B. Saunders, 1986.

Murphy GE, Wetzel RD. Suicide risk by birth cohort in the United States 1949–1974. *Archives of General Psychiatry* 37:519–523, 1980.

Muscat JE. Characteristics of childhood homicide in Ohio, 1974–1984. *American Journal of Public Health* 78:822–824, 1988.

National Center for Health Statistics. *Vital Statistics of the United States, 1960–1979.* Washington, DC: U.S. Government Printing Office, 1964–1983.

National Center for Health Statistics. *Annual Summary for the United States, 1979.* Monthly Vital Statistics Report, Vol. 28, No. 13. DHHS Pub. No. (PHS) 81-1120. Hyattsville, MD: U.S. Public Health Service, 1980.

National Center for Health Statistics. *Advance Report of Final Mortality Statistics, 1989.* Monthly Vital Statistics Report, Vol. 40, No. 8, Suppl. 2. Hyattsville, MD: U.S. Public Health Service, 1992.

National Center for Injury Prevention and Control. *The Prevention of Youth Violence: A Framework for Community Action.* Atlanta: Centers for Disease Control, 1993.

National Commission on Correctional Health Care. *Report of the Committee on Juvenile Health.* Chicago: National Commission on Correctional Health Care, 1991.

Novick J. Attempted suicide in adolescence: The suicide sequence. In *Suicide in the Young* (Sudak HS, Ford AB, Rushforth NB, eds.). Boston: John Wright/PSG, 1984.

O'Carroll PW. Homicides among black males 15–24 years of age, 1970–1984. *Morbidity and Mortality Weekly Reports* 37 (Suppl. S-1):53–60, 1988.

Offer D, Ostrov E, Howard KI, Atkinson R. *The Teenage World: Adolescents' Self-Image in Ten Countries.* New York: Plenum, 1988.

Offer D, Schonert-Reichl KA. Debunking the myths of adolescence: Findings from recent research. *Journal of the American Academy of Child and Adolescent Psychiatry* 31:1003–1014, 1992.

Olds DL, Kitzman H. Can home visitation improve the health of women and children at environmental risk? *Pediatrics* 86:108–116, 1990.

Paget KF, Noam GG, Borst S. Ego development, psychiatric diagnoses, and gender in adolescence: A developmental psychopathology study. Paper presented at the Annual Meeting of the American Psychological Society, Dallas, TX, June 1990.

Palmer S, Humphrey J. Criminal homicide followed by offender's suicide. *Suicide and Life-Threatening Behavior* 10:106–118, 1980.

Pfeffer CR (ed.). *Suicide among Youth: Perspectives on Risk and Prevention.* Washington, DC: American Psychiatric Press, 1989.

Phillips DP. Suicide, motor vehicle fatalities, and the mass media. *American Journal of Sociology* 84:1150–1174, 1979.

Phillips DP. The impact of fictional television stories on U.S. adult fatalities. *American Journal of Sociology* 87:1340–1359, 1982.

Phillips DP, Carstensen LL. Clustering of teenager suicides after television news stories about suicide. *New England Journal of Medicine* 315:684–689, 1986.

Phillips DP, Paight DJ. The impact of televised movies about suicide. *New England Journal of Medicine* 317:809–811, 1987.

Pine F. *Drive, Ego, Object, and Self.* New York: Basic Books, 1990.

Prescott JW. Body pleasure and the origins of violence. *Bulletin of the Atomic Scientists,* pp. 10–20, November 1975.

Prothrow-Stith D. Interdisciplinary intervention applicable to prevention of interpersonal violence and homicide in black youth. In *Report of the Secretary's Task Force on Black and Minority Health. Vol. 5: Homicide, Suicide, and Unintentional Injuries.* Washington, DC: U.S. Government Printing Office, 1986.

Pynoos R, Eth S. Developmental perspectives on psychic trauma in childhood. In *Trauma and Its Wake* (Figley CR, ed.). New York: Brunner/Mazel, 1985.

Pynoos RS, Nader K. Psychological first aid and treatment approach to children exposed to community violence: Research implications. *Journal of Traumatic Stress* 1(4):445–473, 1988.

Pynoos RS, Nader K. Children's exposure to violence and traumatic death. *Psychiatric Annals* 20(6):334–344, 1990.

Reiser DE. Self psychology and the problem of suicide. In *Progress in Self Psychology,* Vol. 2 (Goldberg A, ed.). New York: Guilford Press, 1986.

Remafedi G, Farrow J, Deisher R. Risk factors for attempted suicide in gay and bisexual youth. *Pediatrics* 87:869–875, 1991.

Report of the Surgeon General's Workshop on Violence and Public Health. Washington, DC: U.S. Government Printing Office, 1986.

Report of the Secretary's Task Force on Youth Suicide, 4 vols. DHHS Pub. No. (ADM) 89-1621 to 89-1624. Washington, DC: U.S. Government Printing Office, 1989.

Rich CL, Young D, Fowler RC. San Diego Suicide Study: I. Young vs. old subjects. *Archives of General Psychiatry* 43:577–582, 1986.

Rifkin A, Wortman R, Reardon G, Siris SG. Psychotropic medication in adolescents: A review. *Journal of Clinical Psychiatry* 47:400–408, 1986.

Rivara FP, Mueller BA. The epidemiology and prevention of pediatric head injury. *Journal of Head Trauma Rehabilitation* 1:7–15, 1986.

Robins E. Completed suicide. In *Suicide* (Roy A, ed.). Baltimore: Williams & Wilkins, 1986.

Robins E, Gassner S, Kayes J, Wilkinson RH, Murphy GE. The

communication of suicidal intent: A study of 134 consecutive cases of successful (completed) suicide. *American Journal of Psychiatry* 115:724–733, 1959.

Robins LN, Helzer JE, Weissman MM, Orvaschel H, Gruenberg E, Burke JD, Regier DA. Lifetime prevalence of specific psychiatric disorders in three sites. *Archives of General Psychiatry* 41:949–958, 1984.

Ropp L, Visitainer P, Uman J, Treloar. Death in the city: An American childhood tragedy. *Journal of the American Medical Association,* 267:2905–2910, 1992.

Rose HM. *Black Homicide and the Urban Environment.* Washington, DC: U.S. Government Printing Office, 1981.

Rosenbaum M. The role of depression in couples involved in murder–suicide and homicide. *American Journal of Psychiatry* 147:1036–1039, 1990.

Rosenbaum M, Richman J. Suicide: The role of hostility and death wishes from the family and significant others. *American Journal of Psychiatry* 126:128–131, 1970.

Rosenberg ML, Eddy DM, Wolpert RC, Browmas EP. Developing strategies to prevent youth suicide. In *Suicide among Youth: Perspectives on Risk and Prevention.* (Pfeffer CR, ed.). Washington, DC: American Psychiatric Press, 1989.

Rosenberg ML, Gelles RJ, Holinger PC, Zahn MA, Conn JM, Fajman NN, Karlson TA. Violence: Homicide, assault, and suicide. *American Journal of Preventive Medicine* 3(No. 5—Suppl.):164–178, 1987.

Rosenberg ML, Mercy JA, Houk VN. Guns and adolescent suicides. *Journal of the American Medical Association* 266:3030, 1991.

Rothberg JM, Bartone PT, Holloway HC, Marlowe DH. Life and death in the US Army. *Journal of the American Medical Association* 264:2241–2244, 1990.

Roy A. Genetics and suicidal behavior. In *Report of the Secretary's Task Force on Youth Suicide. Vol. 2: Risk Factors for Youth Suicide.* DHHS Pub. No. (ADM) 89-1622. Washington, DC: U.S. Government Printing Office.

Runeson B. Mental disorder in youth suicide. *Acta Psychiatric Scandinavica* 79:490–497, 1989.

Runyan CW, Gerken EA. Epidemiology and prevention of adolescent injury. *Journal of the American Medical Association* 262:2273–2279, 1989.

Rutter M. Psychological therapies in child psychiatry: Issues and prospects. In *Modern Child Psychiatry* (Hersov L, Rutter M, eds.). Oxford: Blackwell, 1986.

Ryan ND. Pharmacotherapy of adolescent major depression: Beyond TCAs. *Psychopharmacology Bulletin* 26:75–79, 1990.

Rynearson EK. Psychological effects of unnatural dying on bereavement. *Psychiatric Annals* 16:272–275, 1986.

Sabbath JC. The suicidal adolescent—the expendable child. *Journal of the American Academy of Child Psychiatry* 8:272–285, 1969.

Schonert KA. Sex differences in moral reasoning among emotionally disturbed adolescents. In *Adolescent Psychiatry: Developmental and Clinical Studies* (Feinstein S, ed.). Chicago: University of Chicago Press, 1992.

Schuckit MA, Schuckit JJ. Substance use and abuse: A risk factor in youth suicide. In *Report of the Secretary's Task Force on Youth Suicide. Vol. 2: Risk Factors for Youth Suicide.* DHHS Pub. No. (ADM) 89-1622. Washington, DC: U.S. Government Printing Office.

Seiden RH. Suicide among youth: A review of the literature, 1900–1967. *Bulletin of Suicidology* (Suppl.), 1969.

Seiden RH, Freitas RP. Shifting patterns of deadly violence. *Suicide and Life-Threatening Behavior* 10:195–209, 1980.

Seven deadly days. *Time,* pp. 30–60, July 17, 1989.

Shaffer D. The epidemiology of teen suicide: An examination of risk factors. *Journal of Clinical Psychiatry* 49:36–41, 1988.

Shaffer D, Bacon K. A critical review of preventive intervention efforts in suicide, with particular reference to youth suicide. In *Report of the Secretary's Task Force on Youth and Suicide. Vol. 3: Prevention and Interventions in Youth Suicide.* DHHS Pub. No. (ADM) 89-1623. Washington, DC: U.S. Government Printing Office, 1989.

Shaffer D, Garland A, Gould M, Fisker P, Trautman P. Preventing teenage suicide: A critical review. *Journal of the American Academy of Child and Adolescent Psychiatry* 27:675–687, 1988.

Shaffer D, Gould M, Traubman P. Paper presented at Conference on the Psychobiology of Suicidal Behavior, New York, September 18–20, 1985.

Shafii M. Psychological autopsy study of suicide in adolescents. Paper presented at the Child Depression Consortium. St. Louis, October 6, 1986.

Shafii M, Carrigan S, Wittinghill JR, Derrick A. Psychological autopsy of completed suicide in children and adolescents. *American Journal of Psychiatry* 142:1061–1064, 1985.

Shafii M, Steltz-Lenarsky J, Derrick AM, Beckner C, Whittinghill JR. Co-morbidity of mental disorders in the post-mortem diagnosis of completed suicide in children and adolescents. *Journal of Affective Disorders* 15:227–233, 1988.

Shakoor B, Chalmers D. Co-victimization of African-American children who witness violence and the theoretical implications of its effect on their cognitive, emotional, and behavioral development. *Journal of the National Medical Association* 83:233–238, 1991.

Silver JM, Yudofsky SC, Hales RE. Neuropsychiatric aspects of traumatic brain injury. In *Textbook of Neuropsychiatry* (Hales RE, Yudofsky SC, eds.). Washington, DC: American Psychiatric Press, 1987.

Singer S. Victims of serious violence and their criminal behavior: Subcultural theory and beyond. *Violence and Victims* 1:61–70, 1986.

Slaby RG, Guerra NC. Cognitive mediators of aggression in adolescent offenders: 1. Assessment. *Developmental Psychology* 24:580–588, 1988.

Sloan JH, Rivara FP, Reay DT, Ferris JAJ, Kellerman AL. Firearm regulations and rates of suicide: A comparison of two metropolitan areas. *New England Journal of Medicine* 322:369–373, 1990.

Solomon MI, Hellon CP. Suicide and age in Alberta, Canada, 1951–1977: A cohort analysis. *Archives of General Psychiatry* 37:511–513, 1980.

Spivak H, Hausman AJ, Prothrow-Stith D. Practitioners' forum: Public health and the primary prevention of adolescent violence—The violence prevention project. *Violence and Victims* 4:203–212, 1987.

Stack S. The impact of relative cohort size on national suicide trends, 1950–1980: A comparative analysis. Paper presented at the 21st Annual Meeting of the American Association of Suicidology, San Francisco, May 28, 1988.

Stedman's Medical Dictionary. Baltimore: Williams & Wilkins, 1966.

Stengel E, Cook NG. *Attempted Suicide: Its Social Significance and Effects.* Westport, CT: Greenwood Press, 1958.

Stern D. *The Interpersonal World of the Infant.* New York: Basic Books, 1985.

Sudak HS, Ford AB, Rushforth NB (eds.). *Suicide in the Young.* Boston: John Wright/PSG, 1984.

Sugg NK, Inui T. Primary care physicians' response to domestic violence. *Journal of the American Medical Association* 267:3157–3160, 1992.

Sulton AD. *National Symposium on Community Institutions and Inner-City Crime: Shaping the Future Agenda of Urban Crime Control Policy and Research.* Washington, DC: Police Foundation, 1987.

Tardiff K. Determinants of human violence. In *Psychiatric Update: The American Psychiatric Association Annual Review,* Vol. 6 (Hales RE, Frances AJ, eds.) Washington, DC: American Psychiatric Press, 1987.

Taylor EA, Stansfield SA. Children who poison themselves: II. Prediction of attendance for treatment. *British Journal of Psychiatry* 145:132–135, 1984.

Timnick L. Children of violence. *Los Angeles Times Magazine,* pp. 6–15, September 3, 1989.

Tomkins SS. *Affect, Imagery, Consciousness.* 2 vols. New York: Springer, 1962–1963.

Toolan JM. Suicide and suicidal attempts in children and adolescents. *American Journal of Psychiatry* 118:719–724, 1962.

Toolan JM. Suicide in children and adolescents. *American Journal of Psychotherapy* 29:339–344, 1975.

Trautman P. Specific treatment modalities for adolescent suicide attempters. In *Report of the Secretary's Task Force on Youth Suicide. Vol. 3: Prevention and Interventions in Youth Suicide.* DHHS Pub. No. (ADM) 89-1623. Washington, DC: U.S. Government Printing Office, 1989.

Truant GS, O'Reilly R, Donaldson L. How psychiatrists weigh risk factors when assessing suicide risk. *Suicide and Life-Threatening Behavior* 21:106–114, 1991.

Turner CW, Fenn MR, Cole AM. A social psychological analysis of violent behavior. In *Violent Behavior: Social Learning Approaches to Prediction, Management and Treatment* (Stuart RB, ed.). New York: Brunner/Mazel, 1981.

Uehara E, Chalmers D, Jenkins EJ, Shakoor B. Youth encounters with violence: Results from the Chicago Community Mental Health Council Violence Screening Project. *Journal of Black Studies,* in press.

University of California at Los Angeles and Centers for Disease Control. *The Epidemiology of Homicide in the City of Los Angeles, 1970–1979.* U.S. Department of Health and Human Services, U.S. Public Health Service, Centers for Disease Control, August 1985.

U.S. Bureau of the Census. *Statistical Abstracts of the United States,*

111th ed. Washington, DC: U.S. Department of Commerce, Bureau of the Census, 1990.

Viale-Val G, Rosenthal RH, Curtis G, Marohn RC. Dropout from adolescent psychotherapy. *Journal of the American Academy of Child Psychiatry* 23:562–568, 1984.

Wechsler H. Community growth, depressive disorders, and suicide. *American Journal of Sociology* 67:9–16, 1961.

Weiss JMA, Scott KF. Suicide attempters ten years later. *Comprehensive Psychiatry* 15:165–171, 1974.

Weisz JR, Weiss B, Alicke MD, Klotz ML. Effectiveness of psychotherapy with children and adolescents: A meta-analysis for clinicians. *Journal of Consulting and Clinical Psychology* 55:542–549, 1987.

Widom CS. Does violence beget violence?: A critical examination of the literature. *Psychological Bulletin* 106:3–28, 1989.

Willie CV. *Black and White Families: A Study in Complementarity.* Bayside, NY: General Hall, 1985.

Williams KR. Economic sources of homicide: Reestimating the effects of poverty and inequality. *American Sociological Review* 49:283–298, 1984.

Wilson-Brewer R, Cohen S, O'Donnell L, Goodman I. *Violence Prevention for Early Teens: The State of the Art and Guidelines for Future Program Evaluation.* Boston: Educational Development Center, 1990.

Wolfgang ME. An analysis of homicide–suicide. *Journal of Clinical and Experimental Psychopathology* 19:208–217, 1958.

Wolfgang ME. Suicide by means of victim-precipitated homicide. *Journal of Clinical and Experimental Psychopathology* 20:335–349, 1959.

Wolfgang ME. *Patterns in Criminal Homicide.* Philadelphia: University of Pennsylvania Press, 1968.

Wolfgang ME, Ferracuti F. *The Subculture of Violence: Towards an Integrated Theory in Criminology.* New York: Methuen, 1967.

Yufit RI. Developing a suicide screening instrument for adolescents and young adults. In *Report of the Secretary's Task Force on Youth and Suicide. Vol. 4: Strategies for Prevention of Youth Suicide.* DHHS Pub. No. (ADM) 89-1624. Washington, DC: U.S. Government Printing Office, 1989.

Zimring FE. Firearms, violence and public policy. *Scientific American* 262:48–54, 1991.

Index